JN125050

歯科学生のための医学英語

第2版

Comprehensive
Medical English for
Dentistry

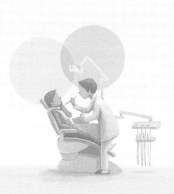

GAKKEN SHOIN

著者一覧

■英文監修

Neil Patel   Senior Lecturer Division of Dentistry
University of Manchester UK

■編　集

影山　幾男   日本歯科大学新潟生命歯学部解剖学第1講座教授

羽村　　章   日本歯科大学生命歯学部高齢者歯科学教授

■執　筆（50音順）

今井　　肇   東京歯科大学教養系研究室准教授

影山　幾男   日本歯科大学新潟生命歯学部解剖学第1講座教授

羽村　　章   日本歯科大学生命歯学部高齢者歯科学教授

壬生　正博   福岡歯科大学医療人間学講座言語情報学分野教授

御代田　駿   奥羽大学歯学部口腔外科学講座口腔外科学分野講師

向井　正太   白鷗大学教育学部英語教育専攻准教授

横山　知美   日本歯科大学附属病院総合診療科助教

吉田登志子   岡山大学医学部非常勤講師

竜　　立雄   RYU矯正歯科クリニック郡山プレミア／元奥羽大学歯学部講師

Asiri Jayawardena   鶴見大学歯学部人文科講師

David Kipler   東京大学医学部国際学科講師

James Hobbs   岩手医科大学外国語学科英語分野教授

Omar Marianito
 Maningo Rodis   徳島大学大学院医歯薬学研究部口腔科学部門
国際口腔健康推進学分野教授

FOREWORD

There is no denying we live in a globalized and international society. This is especially true in the world of medicine, education and research. International research meetings now often stipulate that delegates present their work in English. Moreover, healthcare has been internationalised with health tourism increasingly common. Newly qualified graduates can expect to see and treat patients who do not speak their native language. Knowledge and understanding of Medical English has never been so important.

My first encounter of the study of Medical English was through attending the 21st JASMEE (Japanese Society for Medical English Education) meeting held at the Nippon Dental University School of Life Dentistry, Tokyo Campus. Books such as this owe their existence to all those who have laid the foundations for the many facets of this important field; many of whom I was fortunate to meet at the JASMEE meeting. I would like to congratulate the authors and contributors of Comprehensive English for Dental Students, who have targeted the text towards the dental community. An area of Medical English which is particularly lacking.

The material in this book will be valuable to current dentists, dental students, dental hygienists, dental nurses and dental academics who need to communicate with their colleagues, teams and patients in English. Those who are going to work in English speaking countries, as well as teachers of Medical English, will also benefit. All learning styles are captured by working through the different exercises in this book which covers a wide range of topics from pain diagnosis to discussing cleft lip with patients.

The authors' expertise in this area is evident in the selection of content and tasks, but it is their passion for teaching and the desire to learners succeed that really shines through. I am positive after reading, and completing the exercises in this book, learners will be more confident and effective when communicating dental terms in English.

Dr Neil Patel
Senior Lecturer
Division of Dentistry
University of Manchester UK

第2版発行にあたって

　学生の皆さん！医学英語楽しめましたか？　2020年7月『歯科学生のための医学英語』を上梓してから，2年半が過ぎました．執筆の先生方，歯科学生や歯科領域を学ぶ学生さんのお陰で，この度，第2版を出版する運びとなりました．この間，執筆の先生方や学生さんから多くの建設的なアドバイスを戴きました．この紙面を借りて御礼申し上げます．今回，さらに新しい執筆者が加わり，「歯科用語」「歯科不安症」「歯科インプラント」の3つの新しい章と，歯科用語に簡潔な解説を付した歯科用語集とが追加になりました．これも先生方の熱意のお陰です．心から感謝申し上げます．

　さて，今日，日本人科学者に変化が現れました．国際学会などで，3S (Silent, Smile, Sleeping) と揶揄されていたこともありましたが，この頃は英語が堪能な研究者が増えてきました．楽天や資生堂，ユニクロなどの企業は企業内言語を英語としました．日本の医学部でも，グローバル化にあわせて英語での授業を格段に増やしています．今後，日本の歯学部でも英語の授業は増えていくでしょう．

　さあ皆さん！さらに医学英語を楽しみませんか．楽しいことは続けられます．卒業後も，楽しく医学英語や英語を楽しむことが出来ればしめたものです．

2023年2月

影山　幾男

はじめに

　現在，日本の歯科学生の医学英語能力は危機的状態にあります．Dr. Omar Marianito Maningo Rodis（徳島大学大学院医歯薬学研究部）の調査によると，日本の歯科学生が医学英語に費やす時間は年間平均60時間です．また，3年以上の医学英語の講義をカリキュラムに導入している大学は29校中5校のみです．一方，日本以外のアジアの歯科学生の医学英語能力と比較すると，アジアの歯科学生は，英語4技能（Reading, Writing, Listening, Speaking）のすべてにおいて，日本人歯科学生をはるかに凌いでいます．歯科学生だけのデータではありませんが，2019年，アジアでのTOEFLスコア比較では，日本は29か国中26位，先進国でのTOEFLスコア比較では，36か国中36位（最下位）でした．私の拙い経験でも，20年前のIADR（国際歯科医学研究会議）では，英語を上手に話せるアジアの歯科学生はほとんどいませんでした．しかし，2年前のIADRの学生セッションでは，原稿無しですらすらとプレゼンテーションを行い，その後の質疑応答にも流暢な英語で応答している学生がほとんどでした．私にとって，衝撃でした．日

本の学生諸君！遅くはありません．今こそ医学英語を積極的に勉強しようではありませんか．

まず，なぜ医学英語を学習する必要があるかを考えていきましょう．

◆グローバル化に対応した英語教育改革が必要

平成 25 年 12 月，文部科学省はグローバル化に対応した英語教育改革実施計画を発表しました．2021 年東京オリンピック・パラリンピック，さらに 2025 年大阪万国博覧会などグローバル化は避けられない状態にあります．医学部では，2015 年に日本医学英語教育学会が医学英語教育のガイドラインを制定しました．しかし，歯学部においては，ガイドラインはもとより医学英語のスタンダードとなる教科書さえないのが現状です．歯科学生の医学英語を向上させる必要があります．近い将来，日本の歯科学生，歯科関係者が医学英語を問題なくこなせる必要に迫られています．

◆歯科医師国家試験に医学英語問題が 1 問以上出題

現在，歯科医師国家試験に医学英語問題が出題されています．当初は設問が日本文で，選択肢のみが英単語という簡単なものでしたが，昨今は設問も選択肢も英文となり，難易度が上がってきています．また，今後，さらに問題数が増えることが考えられます．歯科学生にとって，医学英語は国家試験の必須科目なのです．

そこで，歯科大学で英語の授業を担当されている先生方にご執筆をお願いし，歯科学生が習得しておきたい医学用語の知識や英語の 4 技能を向上させる，歯科に特化したテキストを刊行しました．

本書は，歯科疾患をテーマにした 13 の章で構成され，各章は Listening Comprehension に始まり，医学英会話の練習，さらに Reading とその設問，さらに Writing も学習可能になっています．Speaking のみ，講義を担当される先生にお任せすることとなりますが，この総合した 4 技能を学習することで，医学英語力を身につけていただければと考えています．英語が苦手な人も辛いと思わず，易しく楽しく学べるテキストを目指しました．楽しみながら医学英語を学習できれば，しめたものです．しかし残念ながら，このテキストだけでは医学英語の実力が完璧とはなりません．本書を入口に，是非，全員がステップアップすることを期待します．数年後，読者の学生が IADR もしくは他の国際学会において，原稿無しで発表し，Native Speaker と自由に活発な討論ができるようになることを夢見ております．

最後に，この言葉を贈ります．Use it or lose it.

2020 年 7 月

影山　幾男

CONTENTS

本書の使い方

　はじめに，Dental Interview と Reading の音声をダウンロードしてください．

■ダウンロードの方法

　QR コードよりアクセスしていただき，利用規約に同意の上，ご利用ください．

http://www.gakkenshoin.co.jp/item/cme2023/

Dental Interview

Exercise 1　Interview questions

　Dental Interview の会話を聴いて，設問に答えましょう．

Exercise 2　Fill in the blanks

　Dental Interview の会話を聴いて，下線部を埋め，会話を完成させましょう．

★イラストの吹き出しに英語のセリフを入れてみましょう！

Exercise 3　Learn the points

　Dental Interview の会話文を読んで，Exercise 2 の答えを確認しましょう．

Key words in the dialogue

　Dental Interview の会話にでてくる医学用語を掲載しました．単語の意味，使い方を覚えましょう．

Exercise 4　Phrases to memorize

　Dental Interview の会話のなかから，よく使われるフレーズをピックアップしました．現場ですぐに役に立つフレーズです．

Reading

　歯科疾患に関する読みものを掲載しました．辞書を引かなくても読めるようサイドメモに医学用語の和訳を付しました．易しいものからやや難しいものまであります．習熟度に合わせて読んでみましょう．音声がダウンロードできます．

Exercise 5　T or F

　Reading を読んで，内容が正しいときは T を，誤っているときは F を記入しましょう．

Column

　Reading に関連したトピックスや，英語が速く読めるようになる，英語での問診のコツなど，歯科大学で医学英語を教える著者らがいろいろな角度からアドバイスします．

Case Report

　症例報告です．診断してみましょう．

Appendix

●歯科医師国家試験既出英語問題

　103 回から出題されている英語の問題を収載しました．試してみましょう．

● Academic Terms

● Glossary of Dental Terms for CMED

　おさえておきたい歯科医学英語の訳語と簡潔な解説を収載しました．知識の整理に役立ちます．

Index

　訳語を併記しました．

1 Dental Terminology

Dental Interview

Exercise 1 Listen to the dialogue and answer the following questions.

Interview questions

1. Why did Ms. Tanaka ask Dr. White?

_____

2. What is Ms. Tanaka majoring in at the college?

_____

3. What is the meaning of Gloss?

_____

4. What is the meaning of Pharyngeal?

_____

5. What is the meaning of Hypo?

_____

6. Why is Ms. Tanaka struggling with medical terminology?

_____

Exercise 2

Fill in the blanks

Listen to the dialogue and complete the following sentences.

> T ： Ms. Tanaka, a first-year dental student at ABC dental college
>
> W ： Dr. White, a 45-year-old British English teacher and dentist

At a dental college

at 10:00 AM

T ： Good morning, Dr. White. How are you doing today?

W ： Good morning, Ms. Tanaka. I'm fine and hope you are doing well too.

T ： Thank you. By the way, would you ____ _____ ___ _____ ?

W ： Of course, What can I do for you?

T ： We are studying medical terminology in a medical English course. I could not understand lots of _____ _____ . For instance, what does the terminology, the glossopharyngeal nerve and the hypoglossal nerve mean?

W ： You are learning the _____ _____, aren't you? The glossopharyngeal nerve is the ninth cranial nerve. Gloss refers to the tongue and pharyngeal to the pharynx. The meaning of the pharynx is throat. The hypoglossal nerve is the 12th cranial nerve. The meaning of Hypo is below or inferior; therefore, the meaning of hypoglossal is the nerve for inferior or below the tongue.

T ： Wow! That makes sense! I've heard that most of medical terminology originates from _____ or _____ . If we learn the meaning of the Latin or Greek roots, can we easily understand the English meaning?

W ： That's right, Ms. Tanaka! You are _____ _____ medical terminology now. But don' worry; it is just the beginning, and it will get better. You are just starting your medical and dental journey. Clench your teeth and bear the pain.

T ： I will do my best, Dr. White.

W：By the way, I can introduce you to a good booklet for dental terminologies. If you need it, I can give you a copy. Here you go.

T：Wow! Thanks very much, Dr. White. I can read a GLOSSARY of DENTAL TERMS for CMED. What does CMED _____ ____?

W：CMED stands for Comprehensive Medical English for Dentistry. I strongly recommend that you read it. I've never seen such a good textbook like this before.

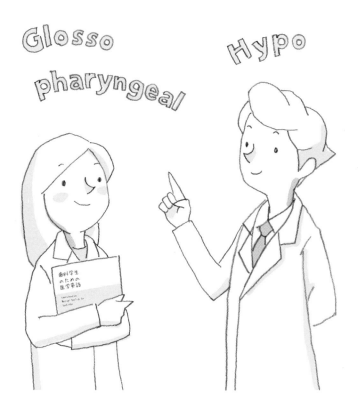

1 Dental Terminology

Exercise 3

Read the dialogue and check the answers.

Learn the points

| T : Ms. Tanaka, a first-year dental student at ABC dental college |
| W : Dr. White a 45-year-old British English teacher and dentist |

At a dental college

at 10:00 AM

T : Good morning, Dr. White. How are you doing today?

W : Good morning, Ms. Tanaka. I'm fine and hope you are doing well too.

T : Thank you. By the way, would you do me a favour?

W : Of course, What can I do for you?

T : We are studying medical terminology in a medical English course. I could not understand lots of medical terminology. For instance, what does the terminology, the glossopharyngeal nerve and the hypoglossal nerve mean?

W : You are learning the cranial nerves, aren't you? The glossopharyngeal nerve is the ninth cranial nerve. Gloss refers to the tongue and pharyngeal to the pharynx. The meaning of the pharynx is throat. The hypoglossal nerve is the 12th cranial nerve. The meaning of Hypo is below or inferior; therefore, the meaning of hypoglossal is the nerve for inferior or below the tongue.

T : Wow! That makes sense! I've heard that most of medical terminology originates from Latin or Greek. If we learn the meaning of the Latin or Greek roots, can we easily understand the English meaning?

W : That's right, Ms. Tanaka! You are struggling with medical terminology now. But don' worry; it is just the beginning, and it will get better. You are just starting your medical and dental journey. Clench your teeth and bear the pain.

T : I will do my best, Dr. White.

W：By the way, I can introduce you to a good booklet for dental terminologies. If you need it, I can give you a copy. Here you go.

T ：Wow! Thanks very much, Dr. White. I can read a GLOSSARY of DENTAL TERMS for CMED. What does CMED <u>stand for</u>?

W：CMED stands for Comprehensive Medical English for Dentistry. I strongly recommend that you read it. I've never seen such a good textbook like this before.

 Key words in the dialogue

terminology：専門用語
glossopharyngeal nerve：舌咽神経
hypoglossal nerve：舌下神経
cranial nerves：脳神経
pharynx：咽頭
struggling with：～に困っている
clench your teeth：歯を食いしばる
bear the pain：痛みに耐える
glossary：用語集
stand for：何の略か

Exercise 4

Phrases to memorize

Let's learn some useful phrases.

1. By the way, would you do me a favour?
   ところで，お願いがあるのですが．

2. You are struggling with medical terminology now.
   医学専門用語に困っていますね．

3. You are just starting your medical and dental journey.
   今，医学と歯学の勉強が始まったのです．

4. Clench your teeth and bear the pain.
   歯を食いしばって，痛みに耐えていきましょう（厳しい医学の勉強に耐えていきましょう）．

5. What does CMED stand for?
   CMED は何の略ですか．

Reading 1

Tooth decay

About tooth decay

Tooth decay can occur when acid is produced from plaque, which builds up on your teeth.

If plaque is allowed to build up, it can lead to further problems, such as dental caries (holes in the teeth), gum disease or dental abscesses, which are collections of pus at the end of the teeth or in the gums.

Symptoms of tooth decay

Tooth decay may not cause any pain. However, if you have dental caries you might have:

· toothache – either continuous pain keeping you awake or occasional sharp pain without an obvious cause
· tooth sensitivity – you may feel tenderness or pain when eating or drinking something hot, cold or sweet
· grey, brown or black spots appearing on your teeth
· bad breath
· an unpleasant taste in your mouth

Seeing a dentist

Visit your dentist regularly, so early tooth decay can be treated as soon as possible and the prevention of decay can begin. Tooth decay is much easier and cheaper to treat in its early stages. Dentists can usually identify tooth decay and further problems with a simple examination or X-ray.

It's also important to have regular dental check-ups. Adults should have a check-up at least once every two years and children under the age of 18 should have a check-up at least once a year.

tooth decay
むし歯, う蝕

acid　酸

plaque　プラーク

caries　むし歯

gum disease
歯周病

abscess　膿瘍

pus　膿

toothache　歯痛

check-up　健康診断

Treatments for tooth decay

Treatment of tooth decay depends on how advanced it is.

· For early stage tooth decay – your dentist will talk to you about the amount of sugar in your diet and the times you eat. They may apply a fluoride gel, varnish or paste to the area. Fluoride helps to protect teeth by strengthening the enamel, making teeth more resistant to the acids from plaque that can cause tooth decay.

fluoride　フッ化物

· Your dentist may discuss a filling or crown with you – this involves removing the dental decay, offering local anaesthetic to numb the tooth and filling the hole.

filling　詰め物

local anaesthetic
局所麻酔

numb　麻痺させる

· If tooth decay has spread to the pulp (in the center of the tooth, containing blood and nerves) – this may be removed in a process known as root canal treatment.

pulp　歯髄

root canal treatment
根管治療

· If the tooth is so badly damaged that it can't be restored – it may need to be removed. Your dentist may be able to replace the tooth with a partial denture, bridge or implant.

Preventing tooth decay

Although tooth decay is a common problem, it's often entirely preventable. The best way to avoid tooth decay is to keep your teeth and gums as healthy as possible. For example, you should:

· visit your dentist regularly – your dentist will decide how often they need to see you based on the condition of your mouth, teeth and gums

· cut down on sugary and starchy food and drinks, particularly between meals or within an hour of going to bed – some medications can also contain sugar, so it's best to look for sugar-free alternatives where possible

· look after your teeth and gums – brushing your teeth properly with a fluoride toothpaste twice a day, using floss and an interdental brush at least once a day

- avoid smoking or drinking alcohol excessively – tobacco can interfere with saliva production, which helps to keep your teeth clean, and alcohol can contribute to the erosion of tooth enamel
- see your dentist or GP if you have a persistently dry mouth – this may be caused by certain medicines, treatment or medical conditions

saliva　唾液

erosion　侵食

GP
General Practitioner
一般臨床歯科医師

dry mouth
口腔乾燥

Protecting your child's teeth

Establishing good eating habits by limiting sugary snacks and drinks can help your child avoid tooth decay. Regular visits to the dentist at an early age should also be encouraged.

It's important to teach your child how to clean their teeth properly and regularly. Your dentist can show you how to do this. Younger children should use a children's toothpaste, but make sure to read the label about how to use it.

Children should still brush their teeth twice a day, especially before bedtime.

How plaque causes tooth decay

Your mouth is full of bacteria that form a film over the teeth called dental plaque.

When you consume food and drink high in carbohydrates – particularly sugary foods and drinks – the bacteria in plaque turn the carbohydrates into energy they need, producing acid at the same time.

carbohydrate
炭水化物

If the plaque is allowed to build up, the acid can begin to break down (dissolve) the surface of your tooth, causing holes known as cavities.

Once cavities have formed in the enamel, the plaque and bacteria can reach the dentine (the softer, bone-like material underneath the enamel). As the dentine is softer than the enamel, the process of tooth decay speeds up.

Without treatment, bacteria will enter the pulp (the soft centre of the tooth that contains nerves and blood vessels). At this stage, your nerves will be exposed to bacteria, usually making your tooth painful.

nerve　神経

blood vessel　血管

The bacteria can cause a dental abscess in the pulp and the infection could spread into the bone, causing another type of abscess.

(https://www.nhsinform.scot/illnesses-and-conditions/mouth/tooth-decay 2022-6-6)

Exercise 5

T or F

If the following sentence is true mark T (true), if it is not true mark F (false).

1. ____ Tooth decay won't cause any pain forever.
2. ____ Tooth decay is not totally preventable.
3. ____ Children should check their teeth regularly by a dentist.
4. ____ The enamel is harder than the dentine, then tooth decay will only occur in dentin.
5. ____ The bacteria can cause a dental cyst in the pulp and the infection may spread in the bone, causing an oral cancer.

1 Dental Terminology

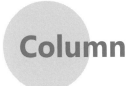

Column

パラグラフリーディングのすすめ

　英語の長文が読めるようになってきたけれど，スピードが遅い．このような場合，パラグラフリーディングという方法があります．ここでは，パラグラフリーディングを紹介します．

　まず，英語のパラグラフ（段落）がどのように構成されているのかを知ることが大切です．パラグラフの構成を熟知できれば，読むスピードは飛躍的に速くなります．ぜひ，パラグラフリーディングを身につけていきましょう．

● パラグラフは以下の３つの部分より構成されている

　1）Topic sentence　　　　（主題文）

　2）Supporting sentence　（詳細説明文）

　3）Concluding sentence　（結論文）

　1）Topic sentence とは，パラグラフのなかで筆者がいちばん訴えたいことです．

　　　通常，パラグラフの最初に置くことが多いのですが，最後に置くこともあります．1 paragraph ＝ 1 main idea がとくに大切で，筆者の主張は１段落に１つです．すなわち筆者が主張したいことが３つあれば，パラグラフを３つ作成することになります．決して１つのパラグラフに３つの主張を含めてはいけません.

　2）Supporting sentence とは，主題文をくわしく説明する文章です．

　　　必ず Topic sentence とつながりがあります．

　3）Concluding sentence とは，Supporting sentence をまとめる結びの文章，もしくは Topic sentence を別の表現で言い換えた文章です．

　　　Concluding sentence が省かれているパラグラフもあります．

● 良いパラグラフには必ず３つの要素（Unity, Coherence, Cohesion）が含まれている

　1）Unity とは統一性のことです．パラグラフ内に Topic sentence と関係ない文章を入れてはいけません．

2）Coherence とは一貫性のことです．パラグラフは首尾一貫して主題文に関連させます．

3）Cohesion とは結束性のことです．文章と文章の間に論理的な結びつきがあることです．

　次ページの文章は第7章の Orofacial Clefts の Reading です．この文章を用いて，Topic sentence, Supporting sentence, Concluding sentence を確認していきましょう．Topic sentence を青色，Supporting sentence を灰色，Concluding sentence をアンダーラインで示します．

1 Dental Terminology

Orofacial Clefts

Cleft lip and cleft palate ("orofacial clefts") are common birth defects resulting from the failure of the tissues to join properly during fetal development. A cleft lip is an opening in the upper lip that can extend into the nose; a cleft palate occurs when the roof of the mouth contains an opening into the nose. Most cases of cleft lip and cleft palate result from interaction of genetic and environmental factors. Orofacial clefts can cause problems with feeding, speech, hearing and frequent ear infections. An ultrasound exam can be used to diagnose cleft lip and cleft palate during pregnancy.

In the developed world, orofacial clefts are present in about one to two of every 1,000 births. Cleft lip is twice as frequent in males as in females, although cleft palate without cleft lip is more common in females. A number of potential risk factors have been identified for orofacial clefts. Babies born to parents with a family history of cleft lip or cleft palate have a higher risk of these conditions, and orofacial clefts appear to be more common in pregnant women who smoke, drink alcohol, or use certain drugs. In addition, some studies indicate that obese women, and women with diabetes before pregnancy, are more likely to have a baby with an orofacial cleft.

Services and treatment for children with orofacial clefts vary in relation to the severity of the cleft, the child's age and needs, and the presence of associated syndromes or other birth defects. Surgery to repair a cleft lip is usually done in the first few months of life and is recommended within the first 12 months of life. Surgery to repair a cleft palate is recommended within the first 18 months of life or earlier, if possible. Many children will need additional surgical procedures as they get older. Surgical repair can improve the appearance of a child's face and might also improve breathing, hearing, and speech and language development. Children born with orofacial clefts might need other types of treatments and services, such as special dental or orthodontic care or speech therapy.

With treatment, most children with orofacial clefts do well and lead a healthy life. Some children with orofacial clefts may have problems with self-esteem if they are concerned with visible differences between themselves and other children. Parent-to-parent support groups can be useful for families of babies with birth defects of the head and face, such as orofacial clefts.

【解説】Orofacial Clefts は 4 つのパラグラフから構成されています．

〈1 番目のパラグラフ〉

　最初の文章が Topic sentence で，口唇口蓋裂の成因に関するパラグラフです．残りの文章はすべて Supporting sentence で Topic sentence と見事につながっています．Unity, Coherence, Cohesion もうまくできています．

　口唇裂および口蓋裂（口唇口蓋裂）は，胎児の発育中における組織の結合不全に起因するよくみられる先天異常です．

〈2 番目のパラグラフ〉

　最初の文章が Topic sentence で，口唇口蓋裂の疫学に主題を置いたパラグラフです．

　先進国では，口唇口蓋裂は出生 1,000 人あたり約 1～2 人に存在します．

〈3 番目のパラグラフ〉

　最初の文章が Topic sentence で，口唇口蓋裂のケアと治療に主題を置いたパラグラフです．ここには Concluding sentence も含まれています．

　口唇口蓋裂のある子どもに対するケアと治療は，裂隙の重症度，子どもの年齢と必要性，関連する症候群または他の先天異常の存在により異なります．口唇口蓋裂を有する子どもたちは，特別な歯科・矯正治療または言語療法のような他の治療とケアを必要とする場合があります．

〈4 番目のパラグラフ〉

　最後の文章が Topic sentence で，口唇口蓋裂の支援に主題を置いたパラグラフです．

　親同士の支援グループが口唇口蓋裂などのような頭頸部の先天性欠損症の赤ちゃんをもつ家族の支えになります．

　いかがでしょうか．Topic sentence, Supporting sentence, Concluding sentence が判別できると，読むスピードが格段に速くなっていきますね．本書に収載されている各章の Reading を，以下のチェックポイントを確認しながら，このパラグラフリーディングを用いて読んでみましょう．

【チェックポイント】

1）各文章のつながりがあるか（Cohesion）．
2）パラグラフのなかにメインアイデアは 1 つか．Topic sentence はどれか？
3）Topic Sentence は効果的か．パラグラフのメインアイデアをはっきり述べているか．
4）ほかの文章はメインアイデアもしくは Topic sentence をサポートしているか．

1 Dental Terminology

パラグラフライティングにも挑戦

　パラグラフリーディングを完全に習得すれば，次はパラグラフライティングになります．パラグラフライティングができれば，論文を書くことが楽しくなってきます．ぜひ挑戦してみてください．

● 良い Topic sentence をつくるキーポイント
　1）Topic sentence は主題となり，パラグラフのなかで最も討議される文章です．
　2）Topic sentence はパラグラフの主文で，筆者が最も述べたい文章です．

● 良い Concluding Sentence をつくる3つのキーポイント
〈最後のセンテンスの役割〉
　1）Concluding sentence は最後に書かれていることが多いため，読者にパラグラフの主題を思い起こさせます．
　2）パラグラフの最後の文章とし，"In conclusion," や "Finally," という前置詞を用いてパラグラフをまとめます．
　3）パラグラフの最後にくる文章のため，読者に次のパラグラフにつながる考えをもたらします（必ずしも必要ではありません）．

● Unity（統一性）& Coherence（一貫性）
　Topic sentence とそれをサポートする他のセンテンスとの密接な関わりが必要です．Topic sentence の周りにはいくつかの文章があり，それらの文章は Topic sentence が主張する主題をサポートします．すなわち，パラグラフのなかの Topic sentence の主題に，すべての Supporting sentences がつながるようになれば統一性と一貫性が認められることになります．

> Remember that besides the topic sentence, a paragraph includes several other sentences which in some way support the main idea stated in the topic sentence.
> If a paragraph announces its main idea in the topic sentence, and if all the supporting sentences contribute to the reader's understanding of the main idea, we say that a paragraph has unity and coherence.

2   Toothache

Dental Interview

Exercise 1   Listen to the dialogue and answer the following questions.

Interview questions

1. How long has Mr. Williams been having pain?

_____

2. Where exactly is the pain?

_____

3. How does he describe the pain?

_____

4. How long does the pain last?

_____

5. What kind of food causes him pain?

_____

6. What is Dr. Gilbert going to do and why?

_____

Listen to the dialogue and complete the following sentences.

W：Mr. Williams, a 45-year-old driving teacher

G：Dr. Gilbert, a dentist

At a dental clinic

G：Hello, Mr. Williams! What seems to be the problem today?

W：Well, I have a _____. It started early in October, so now it's been over two weeks. After I eat, one of my upper teeth on the back right hurts, but not always.

G：Okay, I'd like to ask you a few questions. Can you describe the pain ____ _____?

W：Eating and drinking cold foods sometimes really hurts, and ____ __ _____, the pain comes and goes.

G：How would you rate the pain on a scale of one to ten, with ten being the worst pain you've ever experienced?

W：About three. As I said, it's not really bad. It just keeps _____ _____.

G：How long does the pain last when you feel it?

W：Sometimes it goes right away. Other times it lasts longer than an hour.

G：Are there any types of food or drinks that seem to trigger the pain?

W：Hmm ... cold drinks or food like ice cream usually trigger it, so I've been avoiding them.

G：Does the pain _____ to other parts of your mouth, to the upper left side or lower right side, for example? Or does it remain around the upper right molars?

W：No, it only hurts on the upper right side.

G：What about if I _____ here? Does it hurt?

W：Ouch! Yes, it does. What do you think it is, doctor?

G：It's your right upper wisdom tooth. I'd like to take some dental and panoramic X-rays to find out if it's _____ or _____.

W：Will it be expensive?

G：No, I don't think so. Your insurance should cover routine X-rays.

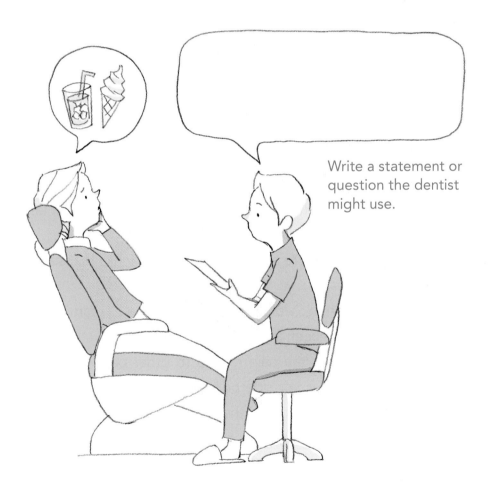

Write a statement or question the dentist might use.

2 Toothache

Read the dialogue and check the answers.

Learn the points

> W：Mr. Williams, a 45-year-old driving teacher
>
> G：Dr. Gilbert, a dentist

At a dental clinic

G：Hello, Mr. Williams! What seems to be the problem today?

W：Well, I have a <u>toothache</u>. It started early in October, so now it's been over two weeks. After I eat, one of my upper teeth on the back right hurts, but not always.

G：Okay, I'd like to ask you a few questions. Can you describe the pain <u>in detail</u>?

W：Eating and drinking cold foods sometimes really hurts, and <u>as I mentioned</u>, the pain comes and goes.

G：How would you rate the pain on a scale of one to ten, with ten being the worst pain you've ever experienced?

W：About three. As I said, it's not really bad. It just keeps <u>coming back</u>.

G：How long does the pain last when you feel it?

W：Sometimes it goes right away. Other times it lasts longer than an hour.

G：Are there any types of food or drinks that seem to trigger the pain?

W：Hmm ... cold drinks or food like ice cream usually trigger it, so I've been avoiding them.

G：Does the pain <u>radiate</u> to other parts of your mouth, to the upper left side or lower right side, for example? Or does it remain around the upper right molars?

W：No, it only hurts on the upper right side.

G：What about if I <u>touch</u> here? Does it hurt?

W：Ouch! Yes, it does. What do you think it is, doctor?

G：It's your right upper wisdom tooth. I'd like to take some dental and panoramic X-rays to find out if it's <u>decayed</u> or <u>embedded</u>.

W：Will it be expensive?

G：No, I don't think so. Your insurance should cover routine X-rays.

 Key words in the dialogue

as I mentioned：私が話したとおり
come and go：現れたり消えたりする
on a scale of one to ten：1 〜 10 までの尺度
keep coming back：何度もやってくる
last：続く
avoid：避ける
radiate：放射線状に広がる
molar：臼歯
wisdom tooth：親知らず
insurance：保険
cover something：何かを抑える

Exercise 4

Let's learn some useful phrases.

Phrases to memorize

1. Can you describe the pain in detail?
   その痛みについてくわしく話してください.

2. And as I mentioned, the pain comes and goes.
   話したとおり，痛みはあったり消えたりします.

3. How would you rate the pain on a scale of one to ten, with ten being the worst pain you've ever experienced?
   1 〜 10 までの尺度では痛みの強さはどのくらいでしょうか. 10 は今まで経験したことのない強い痛みです.

4. Does the pain radiate to other parts of your mouth?
   痛みは口のほかの場所に広がりますか.

2 Toothache

Reading 2

Toothache

About toothache

Toothache refers to pain in and around the teeth and jaws that's usually caused by tooth decay. You may feel toothache in many ways. It can come and go or be constant. Eating or drinking can make the pain worse, particularly if the food or drink is hot or cold. The pain can also be mild or severe. It may feel "sharp" and start suddenly. It can be worse at night, particularly when you're lying down. A lost filling or broken tooth can sometimes start the pain.

It can also sometimes be difficult to decide whether the pain is in your upper or lower teeth. When a lower molar tooth is affected, the pain can often feel like it's coming from the ear. Toothache in other upper teeth may feel like it's coming from the sinuses, the small, air-filled cavities behind your cheekbones and forehead. The area of your jaw close to the infected tooth may also be sore and tender to touch. It's also possible for periodontal disease to give rise to a "dull" pain. Periodontal disease is a bacterial infection that affects the soft and hard structures that support the teeth.

What causes toothache?

Toothache occurs when the innermost layer of the tooth (dental pulp) becomes inflamed. The pulp is made up of sensitive nerves and blood vessels. Dental pulp can become inflamed as a result of:

- tooth decay – this leads to holes (cavities) forming in the hard surface of the tooth

tooth decay　う蝕

filling　充填物

molar tooth　大臼歯

sinus(es)
洞, 副鼻腔（上顎洞）

cavity
空洞, 窩洞, う窩

infected tooth
感染歯

sore　痛む, 痛み

periodontal disease
歯周病

dull pain　鈍い痛み

dental pulp　歯髄

inflamed
炎症を起こした

blood vessel　血管

20

- a cracked tooth – the crack is often so small that it can't be seen with the naked eye
- loose or broken fillings
- receding gums – where the gums shrink (contract) to expose softer, more sensitive parts of the tooth root
- periapical abscess – a collection of pus at the end of the tooth caused by a bacterial infection

There are a number of other conditions that can cause pain similar to toothache, even though the pulp isn't affected. These include:

- periodontal abscess – a collection of pus in the gums caused by a bacterial infection
- ulcers on your gums
- sore or swollen gums around a tooth that's breaking through – for example, when your wisdom teeth start to come through
- sinusitis – which sometimes causes pain around the upper jaw
- an injury to the joint that attaches the jaw to the skull (temporomandibular joint)

Babies can also experience discomfort when their teeth start to develop. This is known as teething.

Preventing toothache

The best way to avoid getting toothache and other dental problems is to keep your teeth and gums as healthy as possible. To do this, you should:

- limit your intake of sugary foods and drinks – you should have these as an occasional treat and only at mealtimes; read more about cutting down on sugar
- brush your teeth twice a day using a toothpaste that contains fluoride – gently brush your gums and tongue as well
- clean between your teeth using dental floss and, if necessary, use a mouthwash

cracked tooth
亀裂が入った歯

naked eye　肉眼

receding gum
後退している歯肉

contract
収縮する, 退縮する

tooth root　歯根

periapical abscess
根尖周囲膿瘍

pus　膿

periodontal abscess
歯周膿瘍

ulcer　潰瘍

swollen　腫れている

wisdom teeth
智歯, 親知らず

sinusitis　副鼻腔炎

temporomandibular
joint
顎関節

teething　生歯

fluoride　フッ化物

dental floss
デンタルフロス

· don't smoke – it can make some dental problems worse

Make sure you have regular dental check-ups, preferably with the same dentist. The time between check-ups can vary, depending on how healthy your teeth and gums are and your risk of developing future problems. Your dentist will suggest when you should have your next check-up based on your overall oral health. Children should have a dental check-up every six months so tooth decay can be spotted and treated early.

dental check-up
歯科検診

(https://www.nhsinform.scot/illnesses-and-conditions/mouth/toothache 2020-6-10)

Exercise 5

T or F

If the following sentence is true mark T (true), if it is not true mark F (false).

1. [ ] The pain in your upper and lower teeth usually comes from the ear.
2. [ ] The inflammation of the dental pulp causes tooth pain.
3. [ ] Softer and more sensitive parts of the tooth root will be exposed as the gums recede.
4. [ ] When your wisdom teeth start to break through, your gums get larger by pressure from within.
5. [ ] You should see some dentists to get a second opinion about your toothache and other dental problems.

Column

"pain" と "ache" の違いは？

「歯痛」を表す英語表現には，"toothache" や "tooth pain" などがあります．この "ache" も "pain" も「痛み」を表す語ですが，ふたつに違いはあるのでしょうか．

Heinemann Dental Dictionary (4th ed.) をみると，"ache" には "A continuous dull fixed pain" という説明があり，連続的で固定した鈍い痛みのことです．一方，"pain" には "A distressing or unpleasant sensation transmitted by a sensory nerve, usually indicative of injury or of disease" というくわしい説明があり，知覚神経によって伝達される悩ましくて不快な感覚のことで，ケガや病気のときに生じる痛みのことです．このように "ache" と "pain" は同じ「痛み」でも，少しニュアンスが違いますね．

英語の表現をいくつかみておきましょう．"ache" は "toothache"（歯痛），"headache"（頭痛），"stomachache"（胃痛），"backache"（腰痛）のように合成語としてよく使われます．"pain" には，"acute pain"（激しい痛み），"sharp pain"（鋭い痛み），"stabbing pain"（刺すような痛み），"dull pain"（鈍い痛み），"throbbing pain"（ズキズキする痛み），"abdominal pain"（腹痛），"muscle pain"（筋肉痛）などがあります（"ache" も "throbbing ache" のように使うことができます）．

ほかにもたくさんの表現がありますが，以下の痛みをネットや辞典などで調べてみましょう．

① gingival pain
② odontogenic pain
③ orofacial pain
④ percussion pain
⑤ pulpal pain
⑥ sinus pain

参考文献：Heinemann Dental Dictionary, 4th edition, Butterworth-Heinemann, 1977

2 Toothache

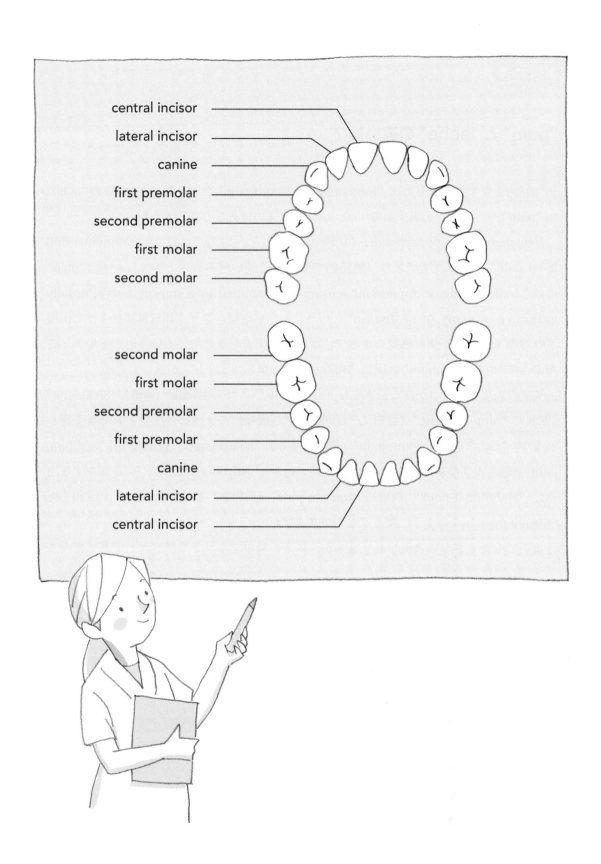

central incisor

lateral incisor

canine

first premolar

second premolar

first molar

second molar

second molar

first molar

second premolar

first premolar

canine

lateral incisor

central incisor

3 Severe Dental Anxiety

Dental Interview

Exercise 1   Listen to the dialogue and answer the following questions.

Interview questions

1. What is the cause of Mr. Jenkins' severe toothache?

   _____

2. Where exactly is his pain?

   _____

3. How does Mr. Jenkins feel while he is in the dental chair?

   _____

4. What does it mean to get butterflies in your stomach?

   _____

5. Why do patients with high blood pressure need to pay extra attention to their health?

   _____

6. What is often used for patients with severe dental anxiety?

   _____

Listen to the dialogue and complete the following sentences.

> J ： Mr. Jenkins, a 30-year-old English teacher from Australia
>
> M ： Dr. Morikawa, a dentist

Mr. Jenkins has a severe toothache. A local dental clinic diagnosed pulpitis (painful inflammation of the pulp) and referred him to the Ochanomizu Dental Center. Today he is scheduled to have his lower left wisdom tooth extracted.

At the dental center

M ： Good morning, Mr. Jenkins. How're you feeling today?

J ： Good morning, Dr. Morikawa. To be honest, I feel really nervous every time I sit in a dentist's chair.

M ： It's normal to feel _____. You can't see what's happening during treatment, which leads to _____. Actually, even I get butterflies in my stomach when I go to the dentist.

J ： I guess we're in the same boat, then!

M ： Exactly. Even patients without _____ illnesses can experience shock from the anxiety and fear of dental treatment. Above all, patients with _____ need to pay extra attention to their health.

J ： I have hypertension and take a blood pressure pill after breakfast every morning.

M ： Did you take your medicine today?

J ： Yes, I did. I hope today's tooth extraction will go smoothly.

M ： Let me check your blood pressure. It's 180/105, which is pretty high. If your blood pressure is high for too long, it can cause serious damage to blood _____, which can lead to various complications. Take a moment to relax, and I'll check your blood pressure in a little while.

Dr. Morikawa checks Mr. Jenkin's blood pressure two more times, but it remains high.

M：Well, Mr. Jenkins, it's been one hour since your first blood pressure reading, and your blood pressure is still 170/95. I'm sorry, but we'll have to postpone surgery today to _____ serious complications such as stroke.

J ：I see. I've been trying to relax, but my body seems to react to the anxiety and fear of surgery.

M：I completely understand. I'd like you to come back to the hospital for the extraction. Next time, with the _____ of a dental anesthesiologist, we're going to give you intravenous (IV) sedation. IV sedation is when a drug is given into a _____ during dental treatment, to relax the patient. The _____ will end within an hour.

J ：I understand. Thanks, doctor. Can I drive on the day of the surgery?

M：No. Unfortunately, you can't drive for 24 hours after receiving intravenous sedation.

J ：I see. OK.

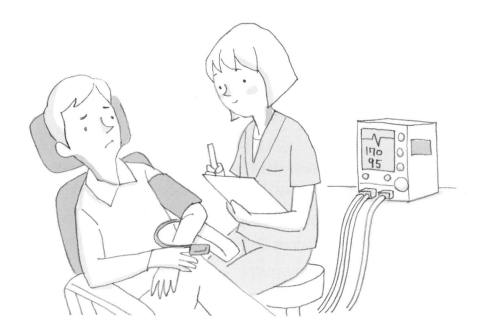

3 Severe Dental Anxiety

Read the dialogue and check the answers.

Learn the points

> J ： Mr. Jenkins, a 30-year-old English teacher from Australia
> M ： Dr. Morikawa, a dentist

Mr. Jenkins has a severe toothache. A local dental clinic diagnosed pulpitis (painful inflammation of the pulp) and referred him to the Ochanomizu Dental Center. Today he is scheduled to have his lower left wisdom tooth extracted.

At the dental center

M ： Good morning, Mr. Jenkins. How're you feeling today?

J ： Good morning, Dr. Morikawa. To be honest, I feel really nervous every time I sit in a dentist's chair.

M ： It's normal to feel anxious. You can't see what's happening during treatment, which leads to nervousness. Actually, even I get butterflies in my stomach when I go to the dentist.

J ： I guess we're in the same boat, then!

M ： Exactly. Even patients without chronic illnesses can experience shock from the anxiety and fear of dental treatment. Above all, patients with hypertension need to pay extra attention to their health.

J ： I have hypertension and take a blood pressure pill after breakfast every morning.

M ： Did you take your medicine today?

J ： Yes, I did. I hope today's tooth extraction will go smoothly.

M ： Let me check your blood pressure. It's 180/105, which is pretty high. If your blood pressure is high for too long, it can cause serious damage to blood vessels, which can lead to various complications. Take a moment to relax, and I'll check your blood pressure in a little while.

Dr. Morikawa checks Mr. Jenkin's blood pressure two more times, but it remains high.

M : Well, Mr. Jenkins, it's been one hour since your first blood pressure reading, and your blood pressure is still 170/95. I'm sorry, but we'll have to postpone surgery today to <u>prevent</u> serious complications such as stroke.

J : I see. I've been trying to relax, but my body seems to react to the anxiety and fear of surgery.

M : I completely understand. I'd like you to come back to the hospital for the extraction. Next time, with the <u>cooperation</u> of a dental anesthesiologist, we're going to give you intravenous (IV) sedation. IV sedation is when a drug is given into a <u>vein</u> during dental treatment, to relax the patient. The <u>operation</u> will end within an hour.

J : I understand. Thanks, doctor. Can I drive on the day of the surgery?

M : No. Unfortunately, you can't drive for 24 hours after receiving intravenous sedation.

J : I see. OK.

 Key words in the dialogue

diagnose pulpitis：歯髄炎と診断する
have his lower left wisdom tooth extracted：下顎左側第三大臼歯（智歯）を抜歯する
get(have) butterflies in my stomach：胸がドキドキする
we're in the same boat：私たちは同じ状況（境遇）にある
chronic illnesses：慢性疾患
have hypertension：高血圧症に罹っている
tooth extraction：抜歯
stroke：脳卒中
dental anesthesiologist：歯科麻酔科医
intravenous (IV) sedation：静脈内鎮静法（アイブイ）

3 Severe Dental Anxiety

Exercise 4　Let's learn some useful phrases.

Phrases to memorize

1. Patients with hypertension need to pay extra attention to their health.

   高血圧の患者は，自分の健康に特別の注意を払う必要があります．

2. I have hypertension and take a blood pressure pill after breakfast every morning.

   私は高血圧で，毎朝食後に降圧剤を１錠飲んでいます．

3. Let me check your blood pressure.

   血圧を測らせてください．

4. I'm sorry, but we'll have to postpone surgery today to prevent serious complications such as stroke.

   残念ですが，今日は，脳卒中のような深刻な合併症を避けるために手術は延期しなければなりません．

5. Next time, with the cooperation of a dental anesthesiologist, we're going to give you intravenous (IV) sedation.

   今度は，歯科麻酔科医の協力を得て，静脈内鎮静法を実施する予定です．

Reading 3

Severe Dental Anxiety

It's fair to say that going to the dentist is few people's favorite thing to do. In fact, over 45% of Britons say they get anxious about visiting the dentist, and almost 12% have such extreme anxiety that they would postpone a visit for a long time, unless it were an emergency. Such people have a dental phobia—even just the thought of a visit to the dentist can lead to horrifying feelings and sleepless nights.

Our previous research found that people with dental phobia tend to have worse oral health and more cavities because of missed dental appointments, poor oral hygiene, and inadequate tooth brushing habits. Oral health is further worsened by smoking, which causes gum disease, and high sugar consumption, which causes large cavities.

Poor oral health can affect people's lives in many ways—especially eating, speaking and smiling. Dental problems can prevent people from opening their mouth in social situations, and broken or missing teeth can make eating and chewing difficult. But, despite this, many people with a phobia will wait until their toothache is unbearable, before they visit a dentist.

A vicious cycle

Patients who put off going to the dentist for a long time are more likely to need more complex treatments, such as root canal treatments, crowns, or surgical extractions (tooth removal). This is because, if a cavity is left untreated, the tooth decay advances and breaks down more tooth structure, thereby exposing the nerve within the tooth (dental pulp), which may then become infected.

Briton
イギリス人

dental phobia
歯科恐怖症

horrifying
ゾッとするような

cavity　むし歯

poor oral hygiene
口腔不衛生

gum disease
歯周病

consumption　消費

social situation
人付き合い

vicious cycle
悪循環

root canal treatment
根管治療

crown
人工の歯

become infected
感染する

As the tooth decay progresses, the tooth can break down extensively—sometimes under the gumline—which makes extraction more challenging. For the patient, this often means more pain after extraction and more time spent in the dentist's chair.

Of course, any treatment for people with dental phobia can induce anxiety, but complex dental work that requires more time in the dentist's chair, and sometimes multiple visits, can be terrifying.

Need for sedation

Some patients with dental phobia will only accept dental treatment if conscious sedation is offered. This can be provided by dentists with the appropriate experience and training. Gas and air (laughing gas) or sedative drugs such as midazolam can help patients feel more relaxed during dental procedures. Some patients may be referred for a general anesthetic, but such drugs must be administered in a hospital.

Unfortunately, specialists and dentists that treat people with dental phobias have long waiting lists. This can leave patients in a difficult situation if they have dental problems or severe pain but feel too frightened to accept standard treatment.

Other ways to help patients

Some hospitals and dental practices are using cognitive behavioral therapy (CBT) to help patients overcome their dental phobia. A study at King's College London found that CBT was highly effective for patients with dental phobia, as it enabled them to overcome their fear of visiting the dentist and to receive treatment without sedation.

We are investigating the possibility of offering more tailored advice on oral hygiene practices, such as better brushing technique and guidance on quitting smoking. The hope is that arming patients with more knowledge will help them feel more confident

tooth decay
むし歯

extensively
広範囲にわたって

gumline (gum line)
=gingival margin
歯肉線

induce anxiety
不安を誘発する

conscious sedation
意識下鎮静

laughing gas
笑気ガス

sedative drug
鎮静剤

midazolam
ミダゾラム
(麻酔導入薬・鎮静薬の
1つ)

be referred for
～を勧められる

general anesthetic
全身麻酔

standard treatment
標準治療

cognitive behavioral
therapy (CBT)
認知行動療法

more tailored advice
個々の状況により適し
たアドバイス

arming patient with
患者に～を与える

in their oral hygiene, which should lower the risk of further disease and reduce anxiety associated with dental visits.

Ultimately, any phobia can be difficult to manage, but when it's a phobia that affects your day-to-day health and quality of life, the effects can be devastating. So, given the fact that some phobias appear to run in families, it's clear that this helps both the patients of today and those of tomorrow.

given the fact that
〜ということを考えると

run in (the/one's)
family
(ある性質が)家族に遺伝している/そういう家系だ

(https://theconversation.com/fear-of-the-dentist-what-is-ental-phobia-and-dental-anxiety-115953)

Exercise 5

T or F

If the following sentence is true mark T (true), if it is not true mark F (false).

1. ____ Almost 12% of Britons have such high levels of dental anxiety that they would avoid visiting the dentist, even if it were an emergency.

2. ____ A study found that people with dental phobias were more likely to have cavities and that their oral health-related quality of life was worse.

3. ____ Dental phobia leaves people feeling completely overwhelmed and terrified by the thought of visiting the dentist.

4. ____ Cognitive Behavioral Therapy enables people with dental phobia to overcome their fear of visiting the dentist and to receive intravenous sedation.

5. ____ Intravenous sedation is an effective way to reduce anxiety in patients and makes potentially stressful procedures more satisfying for them.

Column

Structure of the tooth
（歯の構造）

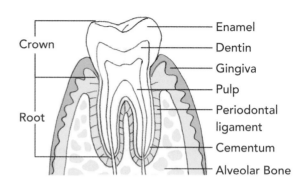

歯はエナメル質（Enamel），象牙質（Dentin），セメント質（Cementum）という3つの硬組織とそれに囲まれた最も内部にある歯髄（Pulp）からできています．歯が口腔内に露出している部分を歯冠（Crown），歯冠より下の部分を歯根（Root）といいます．歯の中心部には歯髄腔（Pulp cavity）があり，歯の神経と呼ばれる歯髄（Pulp）が通っています．歯にかかる衝撃を受け止め，顎にかかる力を吸収・緩和するために，歯根部分の表面と歯槽骨は歯根膜という線維性の結合組織で結びついています．歯は歯槽骨，歯肉，歯根膜の支持組織によって支えられています．

① **エナメル質**（Enamel）：歯の表面部分で人間のからだのなかで一番硬いといわれ，2〜3mm くらいの厚みがあります．

② **象牙質**（Dentin）：歯の二層目部分で，エナメル質より軟らかく，黄色みのある部分です．むし歯が象牙質まで達すると痛みが急速に広がります．

③ **歯髄**［**歯の神経**］（Dental pulp）：歯の中央部分で，神経や血管が含まれる部分です．歯に栄養や酸素を送ります．むし歯が歯髄まで達すると痛みが強くなります．

④ **セメント質**（Cementum）：歯根の表面を覆う部分です．

⑤ **歯肉**（Gums/Gingiva）：歯茎のことで，歯槽骨をつなぎとめ，保護している部分です．歯肉炎を起こすと出血がみられます．

⑥ **歯槽骨**（Alveolar Bone）：歯を支える顎の骨です．歯周病が進行すると，歯槽骨の支えがなくなり，歯がグラグラ動いたりして歯の脱落につながります．

⑦ **歯根膜**（Periodontal Membrane/Periodontal Ligament）：歯槽骨と歯をつなぐ薄い膜です．「硬い」，「軟らかい」などの嚙みごたえを感じ，歯や歯槽骨にかかる嚙む力を調節するクッションの役割をしています．

4   Oral Hygiene

Dental Interview

Exercise 1   Listen to the dialogue and answer the following questions.

Interview questions

1. When did Mr. Brown have his last dental check-up?

   _____

2. Has he had any serious disorder before?

   _____

3. What kind of problem does he have?

   _____

4. What is Dr. Yamada's recommendation?

   _____

5. How many times should he visit a dental clinic?

   _____

Listen to the dialogue and complete the following sentences.

Fill in the blanks

> B : Mr. Brown, a 55-year-old man
> Y : Dr. Yamada, a dentist

At ABC dental clinic

Y : Good morning, Mr. Brown. What brings you here today? Do you have any _____ ?

B : Good morning, Dr. Yamada. I have not had a dental _____ for 5 years. I would like to have one.

Y : I see. Is there anything you're worried about?

B : Nothing. I have never had a serious illness before.

Y : Okay. Well, I'm going to check your whole mouth.

After the dental check-up

Y : I'm going to explain the result of your oral examination.

B : Yes, please.

Y : You do not have any decayed teeth or serious gum disease at present. However, due to your _____ _____ _____, dental plaque and tartar have accumulated around your teeth.

B : I see.

Y : Your condition is not severe at this time, but if left untreated, you may develop periodontal disease in the future. We use our mouth daily to carry out multiple functions such as talking, eating and so on. There is not a single day that we don't use our mouth. Additionally, the mouth and the body are related to each other, having good oral hygiene is essential for _____ the body's overall health.

B : What do you recommend me to do?

Y : It is very good that you had a dental check-up. It would have been too late if a disease had progressed. For the moment, you need an appointment to remove the dental plaque and tartar, which cannot be removed by brushing at home every day. I suggest you get regular dental check-ups to keep your teeth and gums healthy. These check-ups also help to detect tooth decay and gum disease at an early stage.

B : OK. How many times should I come?

Y : In general, you should visit a dental clinic _____ a year.

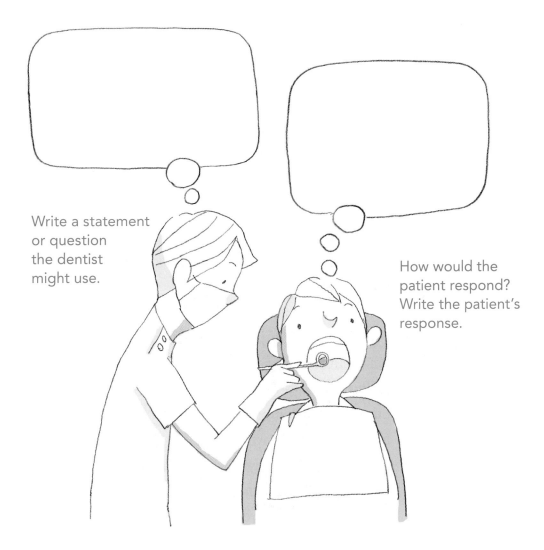

Write a statement or question the dentist might use.

How would the patient respond? Write the patient's response.

Exercise 3

Read the dialogue and check the answers.

Learn the points

> B : Mr. Brown, a 55-year-old man
> Y : Dr. Yamada, a dentist

At ABC dental clinic

Y : Good morning, Mr. Brown. What brings you here today? Do you have any problems?

B : Good morning, Dr. Yamada. I have not had a dental check-up for 5 years. I would like to have one.

Y : I see. Is there anything you're worried about?

B : Nothing. I have never had a serious illness before.

Y : Okay. Well, I'm going to check your whole mouth.

After the dental check-up

Y : I'm going to explain the result of your oral examination.

B : Yes, please.

Y : You do not have any decayed teeth or serious gum disease at present. However, due to your poor oral hygiene, dental plaque and tartar have accumulated around your teeth.

B : I see.

Y : Your condition is not severe at this time, but if left untreated, you may develop periodontal disease in the future. We use our mouth daily to carry out multiple functions such as talking, eating and so on. There is not a single day that we don't use our mouth. Additionally, the mouth and the body are related to each other, having good oral hygiene is essential for maintaining the body's overall health.

B : What do you recommend me to do?

Y : It is very good that you had a dental check-up. It would have been too late if a disease had progressed. For the moment, you need an appointment to remove the dental plaque and tartar, which cannot be removed by brushing at home every day. I suggest you get regular dental check-ups to keep your teeth and gums healthy. These check-ups also help to detect tooth decay and gum disease at an early stage.

B：OK. How many times should I come?

Y：In general, you should visit a dental clinic <u>twice</u> a year.

 Key words in the dialogue

oral hygiene：口腔衛生
dental check-up：歯科検診
decayed teeth：むし歯
gum disease：歯肉疾患（歯茎の病気）
dental plaque：デンタルプラーク，歯垢
tartar：歯石
periodontal disease：歯周病
early stage：早期

Exercise 4

Let's learn some useful phrases.

Phrases to memorize

1. Do you have any problems?
   どうかされましたか.

2. What do you recommend me to do?
   何がおすすめでしょうか.

3. twice a year
   年に 2 回. "once" "twice" "three times" "four times" といった回数を表す副詞を使って頻度を表しています. また, "every" を使って "once every four months"「4 か月に 1 回」のように表現することもできます.

Reading 4

Oral Health

The World Health Organization define health as a state of complete physical, mental and social well-being and not merely the absence of disease or infirmity. It means that we consider health as the environment surrounding an individual. As we are facing an aging society, healthcare systems must find approaches to solve future problems associated with an aging population. From this point of view, we must consider oral health as a global issue.

It is said that oral and general health are closely related. For example, research shows that poor oral hygiene increases the risk of aspiration pneumonia. Insufficient chewing can lead to malnutrition and reduce the quality of life. Periodontal disease is a risk factor for diabetes mellitus and low birth weight. In other words, maintaining a good oral health is essential for one's overall health.

What is the role of dentists? It is important not only to treat caries and perform root canal treatment, to extract teeth that cannot be preserved, to make prostheses, but also to improve oral hygiene. Some patients often overlook or underestimate the importance of good oral hygiene. Dentists can be a good influence on these patients.

Therefore, to approach the individual and society comprehensively, dentists shall prevent disease and perform health guidance in a clinic. Moreover, they should act for the general public and make an environment for health education.

infirmity　病弱, 虚弱

oral hygiene
口腔衛生

aspiration pneumonia
誤嚥性肺炎

chewing　咀嚼

malnutrition
栄養失調

periodontal disease
歯周病

diabetes mellitus
糖尿病

caries　むし歯

root canal treatment
根管治療

extract teeth
抜歯する

prostheses
人工装具, 補綴物

prevent
予防する, 防ぐ

Exercise 5

T or F

If the following sentence is true mark T (true), if it is not true mark F (false).

1. ☐ WHO defines that health is only the absence of disease and infirmity.
2. ☐ The health condition of the whole body is related to oral cavity.
3. ☐ Dentists treat only adult patients.
4. ☐ Dentists should promote and improve public health.
5. ☐ Dentists should perform only health guidance.

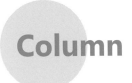

Column

歯科医師と患者のあいだには

　歯科医師の仕事は，むし歯を治すことだけではありません．予防のための歯磨き指導もその仕事の1つです．これは一見して簡単にみえますが，歯磨きを十分に行うのは難しく専門家の指導が必要です．しかし，毎日当たり前にやっていることなので，患者自身のモチベーションはあまり高くありません．では，どうすればモチベーションを高めることができるでしょうか．

　それには一般的な人間関係と同じく，コミュニケーションが重要です．患者さんは，歯科医師とのあいだに立場の違いを感じていることが少なくありません．その隔たりの要因には，立場の違いに加えて歯科医師が用いる専門用語があると考えられます．学校で習った専門用語をそのまま口にして説明しても，それが理解へと繋がることは難しく，かえって障壁となってしまいます．日常生活で使うような平易な言葉で語りかける必要があるのです．

　たとえば，むし歯を取り除いたあと，『歯冠修復物』を装着しますが，その表現ではピンとこない方もいるでしょう．患者さんがわかるように，「ちゃんと噛めるように『詰め物』を入れます」と言い換えるとよいでしょう．さらにその患者さんが外国人で，国際公用語である英語を用いるときに，専門的な医学英語を患者さんが理解できるでしょうか．もちろん，英語でも日常会話と同じような説明が必要となるのです．専門用語だけでなく，日常生活で使っている言葉で語りかけることが必要です．そのためには，日本語だけでなく英語の語彙の幅を広げる力を養わなければならないでしょう．

〈Example〉

crown ⇒ cap

caries ⇒ cavity

calculus ⇒ tartar

posterior teeth ⇒ back teeth

参考文献：松久保隆，八重垣健ほか監修：口腔衛生学 2016，一世出版，2016
安井利一・宮崎秀夫ほか編：口腔保健・予防歯科学，医歯薬出版，2017

5 | **Periodontal Disease**

Dental Interview

Exercise 1   Listen to the dialogue and answer the following questions.

Interview questions

1. What symptoms does he have?

_____

2. What explanation did he receive from a dentist he had seen before?

_____

3. What does he think might be causing his symptoms?

_____

4. What kind of medicines did the dentist prescribe?

_____

5. What is the dentist's recommendation after treatment?

_____

Exercise 2

Listen to the dialogue and complete the following sentences.

Fill in the blanks

> B : Mr. Black, English teacher from Canada
>
> K : Dr. Kawaguchi, a dentist

At a dental clinic

K : What seems to be the problem?

B : My gums are swollen.

K : When did the _____ start?

B : About 1month ago, it started to feel swollen.

K : Do you know where?

B : It is the upper left side, at the back.

K : Is there any _____?

B : It bleeds every time I brush my teeth.

K : Do you have any pain?

B : Not so much, but it feels a bit _____.

K : Did this happen before?

B : Yes, I felt my tooth was a little bit loose before I went to a dentist.

K : What _____ did you get?

B : The dentist told me that I had _____ disease. I had my teeth cleaned and was given brushing instructions.

K : I see. Did your symptoms get better at that time?

B : Yes, I brushed it carefully then the symptoms eased gradually.

K : Did you see a dentist after your gum swelling started this time?

B : No.

K : Do you have any _____ why you have such symptoms?

B : I think it might be because I've been busy these days and haven't brushed enough.

K : I see. Then I will examine your teeth.

The result of the examination revealed that he suffered from progressive periodontal disease. The surgery for reducing periodontal pocketing was performed.

After the treatment

K : Well, that's it Mr. Black! Please be careful not to _____ your cheeks or lips, because your mouth is still _____. I'm going to give you ___ _____ for painkillers, antibiotics and stomach medicine. You can take it to the _____ in the next building. Take the painkiller and stomach medicine if you have severe pain; otherwise, you don't need to take them. Take the _____ for at least three days. If you have any problems, please give us a call right away, even at night.

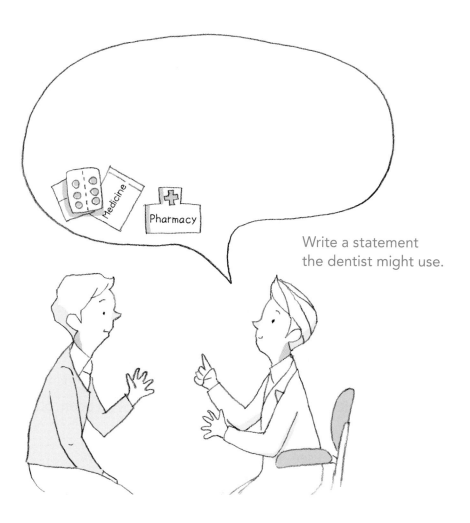

Write a statement the dentist might use.

5 Periodontal Disease

Read the dialogue and check the answers.

Learn the points

> B : Mr. Black, English teacher from Canada
> K : Dr. Kawaguchi, a dentist

At a dental clinic

K : What seems to be the problem?

B : My gums are swollen.

K : When did the <u>swelling</u> start?

B : About 1month ago, it started to feel swollen.

K : Do you know where?

B : It is the upper left side, at the back.

K : Is there any <u>bleeding</u>?

B : It bleeds every time I brush my teeth.

K : Do you have any pain?

B : Not so much, but it feels a bit <u>loose</u>.

K : Did this happen before?

B : Yes, I felt my tooth was a little bit loose before I went to a dentist.

K : What <u>explanation</u> did you get?

B : The dentist told me that I had <u>gum</u> disease. I had my teeth cleaned and was given brushing instructions.

K : I see. Did your symptoms get better at that time?

B : Yes, I brushed it carefully then the symptoms eased gradually.

K : Did you see a dentist after your gum swelling started this time?

B : No.

K : Do you have any <u>idea</u> why you have such symptoms?

B : I think it might be because I've been busy these days and haven't brushed enough.

K : I see. Then I will examine your teeth.

The result of the examination revealed that he suffered from progressive periodontal disease. The surgery for reducing periodontal pocketing was performed.

After the treatment

K：Well, that's it Mr. Black! Please be careful not to <u>bite</u> your cheeks or lips, because your mouth is still <u>numb</u>. I'm going to give you <u>a prescription</u> for painkillers, antibiotics and stomach medicine. You can take it to the <u>pharmacy</u> in the next building. Take the painkiller and stomach medicine if you have severe pain; otherwise, you don't need to take them. Take the <u>antibiotics</u> for at least three days. If you have any problems, please give us a call right away, even at night.

 Key words in the dialogue

periodontal disease：歯周病
swelling（名）：腫脹，（形）腫れている
bleeding：出血
loose：（歯が）浮いている，ぐらついた
ease（動）：（症状などが）楽になる，和らぐ，（名）平易，楽
examine：診察する，検査する
numb：痺れる．麻痺している．
prescription：処方箋
antibiotics：抗菌薬

Exercise 4

Let's learn some useful phrases.

Phrases to memorize

1. Do you have any idea why you have such symptoms?
   なぜこのような症状があるのか思い当たりますか？

2. Please be careful not to bite your cheeks or lips, because your mouth is still numb.
   まだ，麻酔が効いていますので，頬や唇を噛まないようにしてください．

Reading 5

Periodontal Disease

What is Periodontal Disease?

Periodontal disease is a disease that originates in periodontal tissue and as a result, the function of the periodontal tissue is damaged. Periodontal disease is an inflammatory disease caused by bacterial infection. Periodontal disease is classified into gingivitis and periodontitis.

Gingivitis is inflammation in which only the gums around the teeth are swollen. If the boundary between the teeth and gums (gum crevice) is not thoroughly cleaned, bacteria stagnate (accumulation of plaque), and the margins of the gums become inflamed becoming red and swollen. This is called gingivitis.

Periodontitis is an advanced disease of gingivitis. When inflammation persists, the boundary between the teeth and the gums breaks down, deepening the gap and forming a periodontal pocket. As plaque further penetrates along this gap, the destruction progresses further. Next, the gum tissue and the alveolar bone that support the teeth are damaged and the teeth start to become mobile. This is called periodontitis.

Characteristics of Periodontal Disease

Gums around the teeth swell, become red or bleed when touched. The gums swell, so the periodontal pocket becomes deeper. Pus may also develop. The gums later recede and the roots of the teeth can be exposed.

Treatment

Periodontal disease can be treated by tooth brushing properly. However, tartar cannot be removed with a toothbrush,

---

periodontal disease
歯周疾患, 歯周病

tissue　組織

inflammatory
炎症性の

infection　感染

gingivitis　歯肉炎

periodontitis　歯周炎

gum crevice　歯肉溝

accumulation
蓄積, 堆積

plaque　歯垢

periodontal pocket
歯周ポケット

alveolar bone
歯槽骨

pus　膿
<small>うみ</small>

tartar (calculus)　歯石

so it must be removed by mechanical scaling. The important thing is to keep the tooth surface clean and free of plaque. In a case of progressed periodontal disease, surgery may be performed to reduce the depth of the periodontal pocket.

surgery　手術

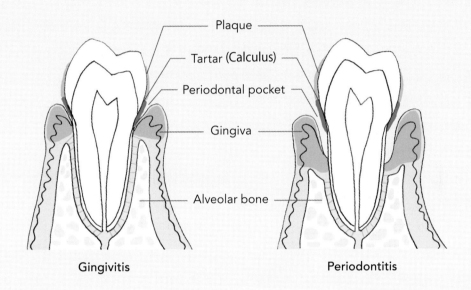

Plaque

Tartar (Calculus)

Periodontal pocket

Gingiva

Alveolar bone

Gingivitis　　　　　　　　　　　Periodontitis

Exercise 5

T or F

If the following sentence is true mark T (true), if it is not true mark F (false).

1. _____ Inflammation confined to the gums is called gingivitis.
2. _____ Both gingivitis and periodontitis are included periodontal disease.
3. _____ If periodontitis is not treated, it can progress to gingivitis.
4. _____ Tartar can be removed with a toothbrush.
5. _____ Periodontal disease can be prevented by routine tooth care.

Column

行動科学のすすめ

　歯周病やう蝕は，生活習慣病です．患者さんのライフスタイルに関連しているため，その治療や予防には患者の自己管理が必要です．つまり患者さん自らが治療や予防に参加しようと考えない限り，その治療は成功しないのです．したがってライフスタイルを改善に導く手立てが必要になります．そのためには生物学的な技術を中心とした治療だけでは改善が難しく，患者との関係性を良好に保ち，患者を動機づけるなど，人の心理や行動などを理解したアプローチが非常に重要になってきます．このアプローチの背景となるものが行動科学です．

　行動科学とは人の心理・社会的，文化的，倫理的な側面を含める学際的な学問であり，患者を単なる生物学的な存在というよりは，全人的に捉えようとします．そして医療現場において使えるような実学を伴うものであることが望ましい姿です．

　たとえば，ブラッシングに積極的ではない歯周病の患者さんへの対応を考えてみてください．歯周病はどれほど恐ろしい病気か，そのままにしておくのがいかに悪いのかなどの説明に特化した対応が頭に浮かびませんか．もちろん患者さんに自分の病気についての知識をもってもらうことは大切です．しかしそれだけで患者さんの行動が変わるでしょうか．ブラッシングに抵抗している原因は何なのか，それは生活環境が影響しているのか，それとも患者さんの価値観が関わっているのかなど，患者さんが問題をどのように捉え，どのようなニーズをもっているのかを把握しなくてはなりません．そのためにはまずは患者さんの話に耳を傾け，患者さんを知ることから始めることが大切です．そうすることで，それぞれの患者さんに適した手立てを患者さんとともに考えることができます．もし患者さんがブラッシングは重要だと思っていても，ブラッシングを行動に移すことに躊躇をしているならば，ブラッシングを遂行できる自信を高めるよう行動科学に裏付けられたスキルを使用し，患者さんが「できるかもしれない」と思ってもらうように方向付けをしていきます．このようなスキルは保健指導において幅広く使用できますし，歯科への不安や恐怖をもった患者さんや指しゃぶりなどの悪習癖をもった患者さんなどにも応用が可能です．

　行動科学には臨床に役立つさまざまな理論やスキルが提唱されています．一度行動科学に関連する本を手に取って，その世界をのぞいてみませんか．

6 Dental Implants

Dental Interview

Exercise 1 Listen to the dialogue and answer the following questions.

Interview questions

1. Why is Mr. White visiting the dentist?

_____

2. What are the advantages of dental implants, as compared with dentures?

_____

3. What patients might be unsuitable for dental implants?

_____

4. How many visits to the dentist will be required to place the implant and crown?

_____

Exercise 2

Listen to the dialogue and complete the following sentences.

Fill in the blanks

W：Mr. White, a 57-year-old high school teacher

K：Dr. Kato, a dentist

At the dental clinic

K：Good morning, Mr. White. What can I do for you today?

W：Good morning, Dr. Kato. I've got a removable denture for a missing upper front tooth. My previous dentist fitted it a few years ago, but now it's loose and moves around when I eat or talk.

K：I see. Let me take a look. Yes, it's your right upper central incisor tooth that's missing.

W：Recently, I read a newspaper article that mentioned that a dental implant is ___ _____ _____ ____ __ _____.
Is that right?

K：Yes, dental implants _____ ____ _____ _____ _____ _____ than dentures. The implant is actually fixed in the jawbone, so it's more stable in the mouth, almost like a natural tooth. However, before I place an implant, I'll need a CT scan of your maxilla to assess your jawbone. You'll also have ____ _____ _____ _____ to be sure you don't have any systemic conditions, such as diabetes or certain blood disorders.

W：Can you explain what a CT scan of the maxilla is?

K：CT stands for computed tomography, and the maxilla is the upper jaw. A CT scan of the maxilla will show the _____ _____ _____ of the upper jawbone around your planned dental implant, which will help confirm if a future dental implant is going to be stable in your mouth.

W：Okay, I understand. Let's go ahead with the necessary tests and exams.

After the CT scan

K : I have some good news for you, Mr. White. Your CT scan and other tests show that _____ ___ _____ _____ ____ ____ _____ _____. So, with your consent, we can get started with placing the implant for your missing upper incisor. I'm afraid the process involves several stages, which means you'll need to make a few visits to my clinic before I finally fix the crown on the implant.

W : No problem. I'm really looking forward to having the implant placed as soon as possible.

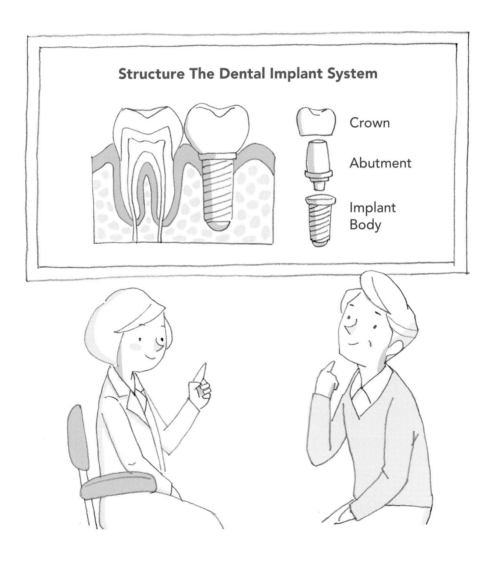

Exercise 3

Read the dialogue and check the answers.

Learn the points

> W ： Mr. White, a 57-year-old high school teacher
> K ： Dr. Kato, a dentist

At the dental clinic

K ： Good morning, Mr. White. What can I do for you today?

W ： Good morning, Dr. Kato. I've got a removable denture for a missing upper front tooth. My previous dentist fitted it a few years ago, but now it's loose and moves around when I eat or talk.

K ： I see. Let me take a look. Yes, it's your right upper central incisor tooth that's missing.

W ： Recently, I read a newspaper article that mentioned that a dental implant is a good alternative to a denture. Is that right?

K ： Yes, dental implants tend to look and function better than dentures. The implant is actually fixed in the jawbone, so it's more stable in the mouth, almost like a natural tooth. However, before I place an implant, I'll need a CT scan of your maxilla to assess your jawbone. You'll also have to undergo some tests to be sure you don't have any systemic conditions, such as diabetes or certain blood disorders.

W ： Can you explain what a CT scan of the maxilla is?

K ： CT stands for computed tomography, and the maxilla is the upper jaw. A CT scan of the maxilla will show the quality and quantity of the upper jawbone around your planned dental implant, which will help confirm if a future dental implant is going to be stable in your mouth.

W ： Okay, I understand. Let's go ahead with the necessary tests and exams.

After the CT scan

K ： I have some good news for you, Mr. White. Your CT scan and other tests show that <u>you're a good candidate for an implant placement</u>. So, with your consent, we can get started with placing the implant for your missing upper incisor. I'm afraid the process involves several stages, which means you'll need to make a few visits to my clinic before I finally fix the crown on the implant.

W：No problem. I'm really looking forward to having the implant placed as soon as possible.

 Key words in the dialogue

removable denture：可撤性義歯
incisor：切歯
alternative：代わり（の），代替
jawbone：顎骨，おもに下顎骨
maxilla：上あご，上顎
systemic conditions：全身状態
computed tomography：コンピュータ断層撮影法，CT 検査

Exercise 4

Let's learn some useful phrases.

Phrases to memorize

1. Dental implants tend to look and function better than dentures.
   歯科インプラントは，義歯よりも見た目も機能も優れている傾向があります．

2. You'll also have to undergo some tests to be sure you don't have any systemic conditions.
   全身状態に問題がないことを確認するために，いくつかの検査を受ける必要があります．

3. I have some good news for you, Mr. White.
   ホワイトさん，よいニュースがあります．

4. I'm afraid the process involves several stages.
   この処置にはいくつかの段階があります．

Reading 6

Dental Implants

A dental implant is a medical device that fuses ("osseointegrates") with bone in the jaw or skull to support a dental prosthesis—such as a crown, bridge, denture, or facial prosthesis. Tooth loss due to injury or disease can result in complications, including rapid bone loss, defective speech, or changes to chewing patterns, and people with missing teeth sometimes feel self-conscious about smiling or talking. Moreover, bite abnormalities caused by tooth loss can adversely affect eating habits, which may lead to health problems such as malnutrition. Thus, use of a dental implant to replace a lost tooth can greatly improve patients' health and quality of life.

Dental implant systems typically comprise an implant body and implant abutment. The implant body is surgically inserted into the jawbone, in place of the tooth root. The implant abutment is usually attached to the implant body with an abutment fixation screw and extends beyond the gumline into the mouth so that it can support the attached prosthesis. Most dental implant systems are made of titanium or zirconium oxide, although other materials are sometimes used.

The final prosthesis can be fixed—i.e., the denture or teeth cannot be removed from the mouth—or removable. In both cases an abutment is attached to the implant body. If the prosthesis is fixed, the crown, bridge, or denture is attached to the abutment with screws or dental cement. If the prosthesis is removable, a corresponding adapter is placed in it so that the two pieces can be secured together.

fuse
結合する, 融合する

osseointegrate
骨結合する

prosthesis
プロテーゼ, 補綴物

denture　義歯

complication
合併症

adversely affect
悪影響を及ぼす

malnutrition
栄養失調

abutment
アバットメント

gumline（gum line）
=gingival margin
歯肉線

titanium
チタン

zirconium oxide
酸化ジルコニウム

Implant success depends on the patient's systemic and oral health. Stresses to which the implant and prosthesis are exposed during normal oral function are also assessed. Ensuring the long-term health of a prosthesis requires careful planning of the number and position of implants, as biomechanical forces generated during chewing can be substantial. Implant positioning is determined by analyzing the positions and angles of adjacent teeth, by laboratory simulation, or by using computed tomography with computer-aided design/computer-aided manufacturing (CAD/CAM) simulation and surgical guides called stents. The long-term success of osseointegrated dental implants depends on the presence of healthy bone and gingiva. Because both can atrophy after tooth extraction, procedures to recreate optimal bone and gingiva are sometimes needed before placing an implant.

gingiva
歯茎, 歯肉

atrophy
萎縮する

tooth extraction
抜歯

Exercise 5

T or F

If the following sentence is true mark T (true), if it is not true mark F (false).

1. ☐ A prosthesis is used to support a dental implant.
2. ☐ A possible complication of dental implants is malnutrition.
3. ☐ The abutment supports the prosthesis.
4. ☐ Biomechanical forces help ensure the long-term health of dental implants.
5. ☐ The success of dental implants requires procedures that recreate optimal bone and gingiva.

Column

読み方を変えながら何度も文章を読む

　英語教育者のあいだでコンセンサスを得ている英文読解力増強法に,「読み方を変えながら何度も文章を読む」というものがあります.

● 文章に書かれている情報を理解して新しい知識を得たり, 内容に共感をする, あるいはその内容をクリティカルな視点に立って深く考えながら読む.

　これは文章の内容の読解に集中をする読み方ですね.

● 文章で使われている語句や文法に意識を向け, 重要な項目を理解し記憶するためにさまざまな工夫をしながら読む.

　この例としては, 辞書をよく読みながら語句の知識を深める, 文章に出てきた新しい単語や熟語のつづり・意味・発音をノートやカードに転記して後で記憶する, 文法的に理解できない箇所について友人や教師に尋ねてみる, などがあります.

● 内容を理解しながら同じ文章を何度も読んで読むスピードを上げていく.

　すらすらと読めるようになるまで繰り返し, 徐々に読解の速度をあげていくという読み方です.

　これらの読み方は, 読解の深さ・正確さ・速さという異なる側面を鍛えるための異なるトレーニングと考えることができます.

　英文の読解については, 人によって読み方に個性が出たり, 同じ人でもその時々で読み方は大きく変わったりということがあります.「今回は読むのは速かったが正確さが欠けていた」,「読解を深くしようとしたために限られた時間のなかで読むことができなかった」,「語彙を調べながら正確に読んでいたと思うが教師の解説を聴いてその文章の複雑さや深さが初めて理解できた」といった感覚に覚えのある人は多いと思います. バランスの取れた安定した英文読解力をつけるためには, 日ごろからこうした読み方の違いを意識し, 読み方に偏りがないように注意することが重要でしょう. 同じ文章を, 読み方を変えて何度も読むというやり方は, こうした点で大きな効果が得られるわけです.

Cleft Lip

Dental Interview

Exercise 1   Listen to the dialogue and answer the following questions.

Interview questions

1. Why is Ms. Smith visiting a doctor?

_____

2. What is a cleft lip?

_____

3. How many babies are born with a cleft lip?

_____

4. What is the doctor's recommendation?

_____

Exercise 2

Listen to the dialogue and complete the following sentences.

Fill in the blanks

> S：Ms. Smith, a 55-year-old housewife
>
> G：Dr. Gregory, a doctor

At a hospital

G：Good evening Ms. Smith. I'm Dr. Gregory. _____ _____ you here today?

S：My daughter just gave birth to a baby girl the day before yesterday.

G：Congratulations! That's great news.

S：Thank you. Although I'm happy to have a granddaughter, I'm also worried because she has a _____ ____. What should I do?

G：Can you tell me a little more? How severe is it?

S：She has a cleft on the left side of her lip. It's about two centimeters long. Do you think I should take her to the university hospital right away?

G：Cleft lip is a _____ _____ of the upper lip that occurs about once in 1000 births. The clefts vary from a small notch in the transitional zone to ones that extend through the lip into the nose. If you are worried about it, please bring the baby with your daughter tomorrow.

S：I will bring them tomorrow.

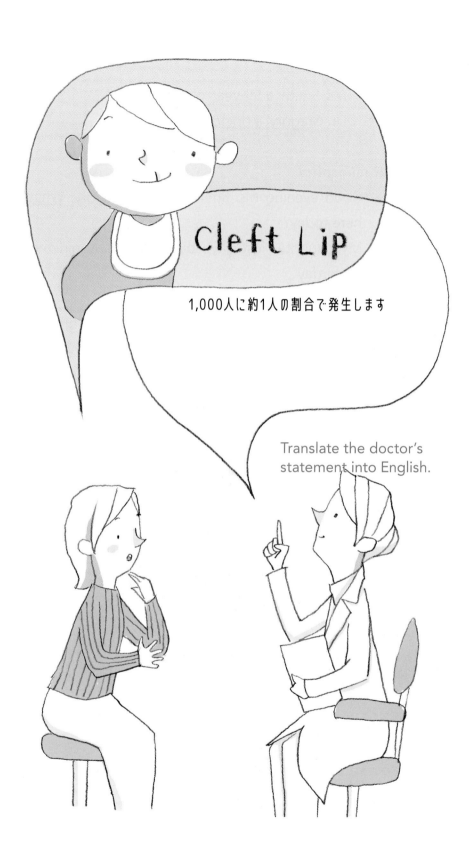

Cleft Lip

1,000人に約1人の割合で発生します

Translate the doctor's statement into English.

7 Cleft Lip

Exercise 3

Read the dialogue and check the answers.

Learn the points

> S : Ms. Smith, a 55-year-old housewife
>
> G : Dr. Gregory, a doctor

At a hospital

G : Good evening Ms. Smith. I'm Dr. Gregory. <u>What brings</u> you here today?

S : My daughter just gave birth to a baby girl the day before yesterday.

G : Congratulations! That's great news.

S : Thank you. Although I'm happy to have a granddaughter, I'm also worried because she has a <u>cleft lip</u>. What should I do?

G : Can you tell me a little more? How severe is it?

S : She has a cleft on the left side of her lip. It's about two centimeters long. Do you think I should take her to the university hospital right away?

G : Cleft lip is a <u>congenital malformation</u> of the upper lip that occurs about once in 1000 births. The clefts vary from a small notch in the transitional zone to ones that extend through the lip into the nose. If you are worried about it, please bring the baby with your daughter tomorrow.

S : I will bring them tomorrow.

Key words in the dialogue

cleft lip：口唇裂
congenital：先天的 / acquired：後天的
malformation：奇形
transitional zone：移行帯（人中の両側）

Exercise 4

Let's learn some useful phrases.

Phrases to memorize

1. My daughter just gave birth to a baby girl the day before yesterday.
    おととい，娘が女の子を出産しました．

2. Do you think I should take her to the university hospital right away?
    できるだけ早く大学病院に赤ん坊を連れて行くべきですか？

3. The clefts vary from a small notch in the transitional zone to ones that extend through the lip into the nose.
    口唇裂は人中の両側の小さな切れ込みから口唇から鼻に延びるものもあり，さまざまです．

Reading 7

Orofacial Clefts

Cleft lip and cleft palate ("orofacial clefts") are common birth defects resulting from the failure of the tissues to join properly during fetal development. A cleft lip is an opening in the upper lip that can extend into the nose; a cleft palate occurs when the roof of the mouth contains an opening into the nose. Most cases of cleft lip and cleft palate result from interaction of genetic and environmental factors. Orofacial clefts can cause problems with feeding, speech, hearing and frequent ear infections. An ultrasound exam can be used to diagnose cleft lip and cleft palate during pregnancy.

In the developed world, orofacial clefts are present in about one to two of every 1,000 births. Cleft lip is twice as frequent in males as in females, although cleft palate without cleft lip is more common in females. A number of potential risk factors have been identified for orofacial clefts. Babies born to parents with a family history of cleft lip or cleft palate have a higher risk of these conditions, and orofacial clefts appear to be more common in pregnant women who smoke, drink alcohol, or use certain drugs. In addition, some studies indicate that obese women, and women with diabetes before pregnancy, are more likely to have a baby with an orofacial cleft.

Services and treatment for children with orofacial clefts vary in relation to the severity of the cleft, the child's age and needs, and the presence of associated syndromes or other birth defects. Surgery to repair a cleft lip is usually done in the first few months of life and is recommended within the first 12 months of life.

cleft lip　口唇裂

cleft palate　口蓋裂

orofacial clefts
口腔顔面裂
口唇口蓋裂

fetal development
胎児の発育

genetic　遺伝的

ultrasound exam
超音波検査

diagnose　診断する

pregnancy　妊娠

obese　肥満の

diabetes(mellitus)
糖尿病

Surgery to repair a cleft palate is recommended within the first 18 months of life or earlier, if possible. Many children will need additional surgical procedures as they get older. Surgical repair can improve the appearance of a child's face and might also improve breathing, hearing, and speech and language development. Children born with orofacial clefts might need other types of treatments and services, such as special dental or orthodontic care or speech therapy.

orthodontic care
矯正治療

speech therapy
言語療法

self-esteem　自尊心

     With treatment, most children with orofacial clefts do well and lead a healthy life. Some children with orofacial clefts may have problems with self-esteem if they are concerned with visible differences between themselves and other children. Parent-to-parent support groups can be useful for families of babies with birth defects of the head and face, such as orofacial clefts.

Exercise 5

T or F

If the following sentence is true mark T (true), if it is not true mark F (false).

1.   All cases of orofacial cleft are caused by genetic defects.
2.   Orofacial cleft can affect hearing.
3.   Approximately 1% to 2% of children are born with an orofacial cleft.
4.   Surgery to repair orofacial clefts is best done when children are older.
5.   Most children with orofacial clefts lead normal lives.

Sources：Wikipedia article (https://en.wikipedia.org/wiki/Cleft_lip_and_cleft_palate)
US CDC (https://www.cdc.gov/ncbddd/birthdefects/cleftlip.html); no copyright
MayoClinic(https://www.mayoclinic.org/diseases-conditions/cleft-palate/symptoms-causes/syc-20370985)

Column

科学論文の読みかたについて

　論文を効率的に正しく読むためには，まず論文の構成を知っておくことが大切です．分野によってその構成は異なりますが，科学論文は一般的に下記の要素で構成されています．

- Abstract（要約・要旨）
- Introduction（緒言）
- Materials and methods（材料と研究方法）
- Results（結果）
- Discussions（考察）
- Conclusion（結論）
- References（引用文献）
- Compliance with ethical standards（倫理的配慮）

　Abstract は，科学論文の多くに設けられ，通常論文の最初に位置づけられています．背景と目的，実験の手法，結果と結論について端的に要約され，内容の全体像が提示されています．全体を事細かに読む前に大まかな内容を把握できるため，論文を読むにあたって予備知識を得やすく，その論文をどのように精読すればよいかを決める一助となるでしょう．

　Introduction は，言葉通り導入の役割を担っています．日本語論文では緒言といいます．研究分野に関する背景が紹介されていたり，論文執筆時における研究の動向や先行研究，それに，その論文を執筆するに至った経緯について記されていたりします．そのような書き出しのあとに，先行研究をもとにした研究分野の課題や今後の展望について触れていることもあるでしょう．とりわけ，科学論文において重要なことは仮説を検証することにあります．Introduction の最後には筆者の仮説，つまりその論文において明らかにしたいことが述べられているため，研究の目的と仮説との関係性について注意深く読み込むことが重要でしょう．

Material and methods では，研究の方法，調査や実験の手法，分析の方法について詳細に示されています．たとえば論文を参考にした人が論文内容を再現できるよう，実験方法や使用した機器・試薬やその供給元などについて明確に記載する必要があります．また，実験の結果や収集したデータに関する分析方法についても紹介されています．

Results では研究の結果がそのまま記載されます．実験を行ったのであれば実験によって導きだされたデータや，その統計が示されています．本文に加えて，数値化されたデータや画像が Table や Figure として描かれることもあります．Material and methods と対になって書かれることが多いため，両者を見比べながら読み進めると，理解が深めやすいかもしれません．

Discussion では，研究の結果を通じてどのような事実がわかったのか，ということを中心に議論が展開されます．ひとつひとつの結果から得られた知見や解釈が記載され，それを補完する他の研究が提示されることもあります．筆者の考えがはっきりと示されていることが多いといえるでしょう．また，研究に関する改善点や今後の展望が示されるのもこの項目です．

Conclusion の役割は，論文をまとめることです．仮説を立てて論証してきた内容を包括的にまとめられているため，著者の主張や論点を再確認することが可能な部分です．

References では，本文中で用いた引用文献などの出典が紹介されます．研究の背景となった重要な論文や研究にかかわる先行研究，比較や考察に用いた論文についても示されるため，ここに記載された論文にも目を通すことで，論述されている内容に対する理解が深まるでしょう．

Compliance with ethical standards では，人を用いた研究などで倫理的な配慮が必要なときには，論文中にその内容を記載します．

上に示したもの以外にも，論文はさまざまな要素で構成されています．ですが，大まかな流れについて把握することは，各々のパートで何を目的としているか読みとるために必要な前提といえるでしょう．

Title から研究分野に関係する内容や興味のある論文を見きわめ，Abstract で全体の内容について理解する．論文の構成要素を念頭においたうえで，それぞれの章を精読し，内容について理解する．そして 10 ページで紹介したパラグラフリーディングを用いて，たくさんの論文を読むことに，ぜひ挑戦してください．

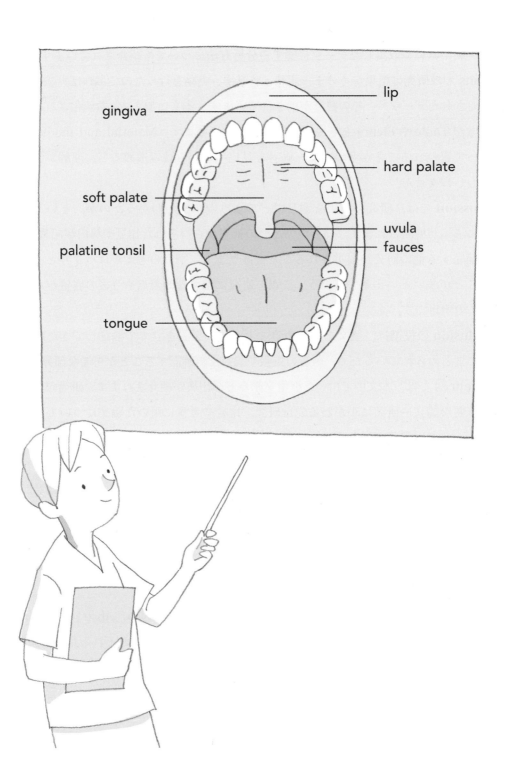

lip

gingiva

hard palate

soft palate

uvula

fauces

palatine tonsil

tongue

8   Leukoplakia

Dental Interview

Exercise 1   Listen to the dialogue and answer the following questions.

Interview questions

1. What is Mr. Brown's chief complaint?

2. What kind of disease has the patient been suffering from?

3. When did the patient start smoking?

4. What is Leukoplakia?

5. What risk factor is associated with lung cancer?

6. What is the doctor's recommendation?

Exercise 2

Fill in the blanks

Listen to the dialogue and complete the following sentences.

> B：Mr. Brown, a 45-year-old American teacher
>
> T：Dr. Tanaka, an oral surgeon

At a dental university

The phone is ringing at 10:00 AM

T：Hello! This is Dr. Tanaka speaking. May I help you?

B：Hello, I hope you can help. I haven't been able to eat for two days because my _____ ___ _____. I also have a white patch on my tongue. Is it possible to _____ _____ today?

T：Did you bite your tongue recently?

B：No, I didn't.

T：All right. Can you come to our university now?

B：Yes.

T：Please bring your medical insurance and clinic cards.

30 minutes later

T：Hello, Mr. Brown. My name is Dr. Tanaka and I'll be treating you today. Before I examine you, I need to ask a few more questions about your _____ _____. Do you have any medical conditions? Have you ever been hospitalized?

B：Yes, I had hepatitis B 10 years ago. I still see the doctor and am on some medication, but I'm in pretty _____ _____ now.

T：Do you smoke?

B：Yes, I've been smoking since I was 15.

T：Let's take a look. Can you open your mouth?

After the examination

T：Mr. Brown. It looks like you have leukoplakia.

B：Leukoplakia? What's that?

T：Leukoplakia is a _____ lesion of the mouth. It can

sometimes develop into cancer. It causes a thick white patch on the mucous membrane of the mouth. I'd like to do a _____ as soon as possible. To reach a definite diagnosis we'll need to remove some cells for examination by a pathologist. Smoking is a risk factor, not only for lung cancer, but also for cancers of the mouth and throat. Try your best to quit, Mr. Brown.

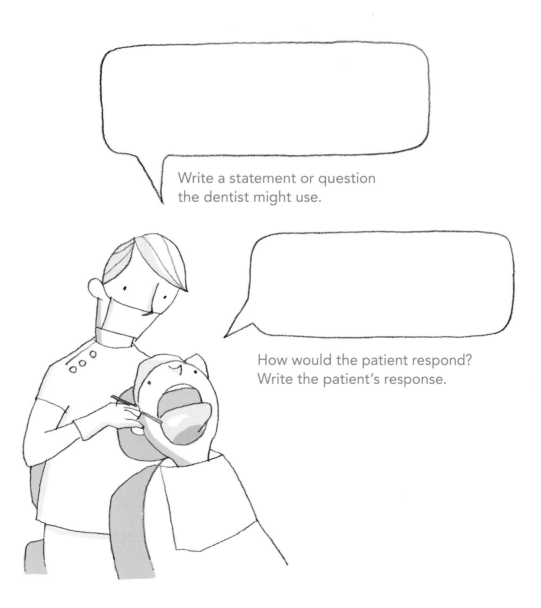

Write a statement or question the dentist might use.

How would the patient respond? Write the patient's response.

8 Leukoplakia

Exercise 3

Read the dialogue and check the answers.

Learn the points

> B ：Mr. Brown, a 45-year-old American teacher
>
> T ：Dr. Tanaka, an oral surgeon

At a dental university

The phone is ringing at 10:00 AM

T ：Hello! This is Dr. Tanaka speaking. May I help you?

B ：Hello, I hope you can help. I haven't been able to eat for two days because my <u>tongue is sore</u>. I also have a white patch on my tongue. Is it possible to <u>get treated</u> today?

T ：Did you bite your tongue recently?

B ：No, I didn't.

T ：All right. Can you come to our university now?

B ：Yes.

T ：Please bring your medical insurance and clinic cards.

30 minutes later

T ：Hello, Mr. Brown. My name is Dr. Tanaka and I'll be treating you today. Before I examine you, I need to ask a few more questions about your <u>general health</u>. Do you have any medical conditions? Have you ever been hospitalized?

B ：Yes, I had hepatitis B 10 years ago. I still see the doctor and am on some medication, but I'm in pretty <u>good health</u> now.

T ：Do you smoke?

B ：Yes, I've been smoking since I was 15.

T ：Let's take a look. Can you open your mouth?

After the examination

T ：Mr. Brown. It looks like you have leukoplakia.

B ：Leukoplakia? What's that?

T ：Leukoplakia is a <u>precancerous</u> lesion of the mouth. It can sometimes develop into cancer. It causes a thick white patch on the mucous membrane of the mouth. I'd like to do a <u>biopsy</u> as soon as possible. To reach a definite diagnosis we'll need to remove some cells for examination by a pathologist. Smoking is a risk factor, not only for lung cancer, but also for cancers of the mouth and throat. Try your best to quit, Mr. Brown.

Key words in the dialogue

a sore tongue：舌の痛み（my tongue is sore）
hepatitis B：B 型肝炎
leukoplakia：白板症
precancerous lesion：前癌病変
mucous membrane：粘膜
biopsy：生検
definite diagnosis：確定診断
pathologist：病理学者

Exercise 4 Let's learn some useful phrases.

Phrases to memorize

1. My name is Dr. Tanaka and I'll be treating you today.
    本日担当させていただきます医師の田中です.

2. Have you ever been hospitalized?
    今まで入院されたことはありますか？

3. I'd like to do a biopsy as soon as possible.
    ただちに生検をしたいのですが.

Reading 8

Leukoplakia

Description

Leukoplakia (loo-koh-PLAY-key-uh) or Oral Leukoplakia (OL) are irregularly-shaped, white or gray, thick, and hard patches commonly found on the gums, insides of the cheeks, bottom of the mouth, and sides of the tongue. OL are generally benign or non-cancerous but there are cases when they become malignant or cancerous especially when they occur together with raised red lesions, called erythroplakia, which may have a high potential for malignant transformation.

Variants

Another form of OL known as Oral Hairy Leukoplakia affects people whose immune systems have been weakened by disease, especially HIV/AIDS. Hairy leukoplakia causes fuzzy, white patches that resemble folds or ridges, usually on the sides of your tongue. Another form of OL is Idiopathic Leukoplakia (IL), which is said to be rare but could be aggressive compared to the common leukoplakia. IL is leukoplakia that is not associated with smoking and is considered as a pre-malignant or a potentially malignant lesion. Another variant of OL is the Oral Proliferative Verrucous Leukoplakia (OPVL). OPVL is also rare, slow growing, and long-term progressive lesion. The etiology of OPVL remains unclear and smoking is not associated with OPVL. Moreover, it is observed more frequently in women and elderly patients over 60 years at the time of diagnosis and it has a high rate of malignant transformation.

leukoplakia 白板症

patch 斑点

benign 良性の

malignant 悪性の

cancerous がん性の

lesion 病変

erythroplakia
紅板症

Oral Hairy
Leukoplakia
口腔毛状白板症

Idiopathic
Leukoplakia
特発性白板症

Oral Proliferative
Verrucous
Leukoplakia
口腔増殖性疣贅状白板症

Etiology

Although the exact cause of Oral Leukoplakia is still unknown, it is believed to be caused by a weakened immune system such as in people with HIV or AIDS, or people who are smokers.

Epidemiology

Oral Leukoplakia usually occurs from 50 to 70 years of age and is twice more common in men than in women. It is also reported that 80% of tobacco users develop leukoplakia.

Symptoms

Oral Leukoplakia generally does not exhibit symptoms and most are reported to exist without pain so most go unnoticed until a visit to a dentist. Thus, it is important to educate patients to report unusual and persistent changes in their oral cavities to dentists.

persistent　持続的な

Differential Diagnosis

Oral Leukoplakia may easily be misdiagnosed as oral thrush or Candidiasis because of its appearance. Oral thrush is a fungal infection caused by Candida Albicans, which is a normal microflora in the mouth. The infection produces white creamy slightly raised lesions that can be sensitive and painful. Like OL, oral thrush is common in people with weakened immune system and those taking certain medications. It is also commonly found in the gums, insides of the cheeks, roof of the mouth, and the tongue. Thus, both conditions can be misdiagnosed easily as one or the other. To differentiate both conditions, it is important to note that leukoplakia cannot be scraped off while oral thrush can easily be scraped off. Another important thing to note is that leukoplakia is generally not painful while oral thrush is, and may produce bleeding when scraped off. Finally, OL does not cause loss of taste while oral thrush can.

oral thrush
鵞口瘡
口腔カンジダ症

Candidiasis
カンジダ症

fungal　真菌

normal microflora
常在菌

scrape off　拭い取る

Treatment

Oral Leukoplakia can be simply treated by removing the source of irritation or trauma with regular check-ups. Other ways include removal of the hardened patches using scalpels or laser removal procedures. Biopsy must be performed to diagnose Oral Leukoplakia at the patient's initial visit.

scalpel メス

biopsy 生検

Exercise 5

T or F

If the following sentence is true mark T (true), if it is not true mark F (false).

1. ____ Leukoplakia is generally benign in nature.
2. ____ Leukoplakia is commonly known as oral thrush.
3. ____ Leukoplakia are white or grayish soft patches that can be scraped off.
4. ____ Leukoplakia can sometimes become malignant especially when they occur together with erythroplakia.
5. ____ Leukoplakia is generally asymptomatic.

Sources：Mayo Clinic & Johns Hopkins Medicine

9   Herpes Simplex

Dental Interview

Exercise 1   Listen to the dialogue and answer the following questions.

Interview questions

1. Why is Ms. Marcy Martin visiting a doctor?

2. What is a cold sore?

3. Has she suffered from blisters before?

4. Are cold sores a curable condition?

5. How can she treat her disease?

6. Can she transmit the disease to anyone else?

Exercise 2

Listen to the dialogue and complete the following sentences.

Fill in the blanks

> M：Ms. Marcy Martin, a 20-year-old college student
>
> T ：Dr. Tanaka, an oral surgeon

At a dental university

T ：What brings you here today?

M：I have _____ on my lips, and it tingles a bit.

T ：Ah, yes. It's a _____ _____; people sometimes called it a fever blister. They're caused by _____ _____ _____ _____ which is very common. Have you ever had a cold sore before?

M：Yes, about two years ago, but this is the first time I have had it checked out.

T ：After you're infected with the herpes simplex virus, it _____ _____ in your nerves. The virus is reactivated and symptoms begin to appear when your immune system is weakened by a cold, stress, or exposure to strong UV radiation for example.

M：Is there any way to cure it completely?

T ：Unfortunately, no. Whenever you have an _____ or _____ _____ on the lips, please come see me as soon as possible. Early use of anti-viral drugs can reduce the symptoms and prevent the spread of the virus.

M：Is it contagious?

T ：Yes. You should avoid all _____ _____ with others until the symptoms disappear. Be especially careful around babies, as the virus can have severe effects for them. The virus can persist for several days, and blisters usually take two to four weeks to heal completely. During this time the virus is highly contagious. Cold sores _____ ____ _____ at the same spot but are usually less severe after the first outbreak. Don't touch the blisters, and be sure to take _____ _____

_____ _____ . That will help them heal faster.

M：Okay, doctor. Thanks very much!

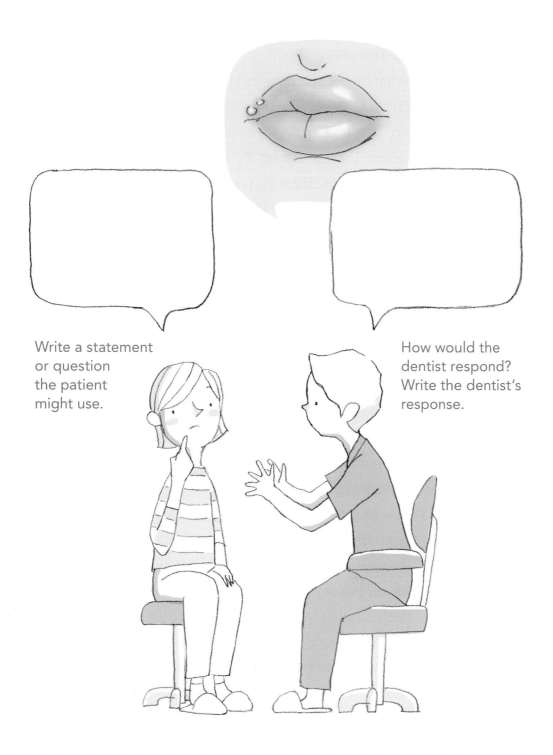

Write a statement or question the patient might use.

How would the dentist respond? Write the dentist's response.

9 Herpes Simplex

Exercise 3

Read the dialogue and check the answers.

Learn the points

> M：Ms. Marcy Martin, a 20-year-old college student
> T：Dr. Tanaka, an oral surgeon

At a dental university

T：What brings you here today?

M：I have <u>blisters</u> on my lips, and it tingles a bit.

T：Ah, yes. It's a <u>cold sore</u>; people sometimes called it a fever blister. They're caused by <u>the herpes simplex virus</u> which is very common. Have you ever had a cold sore before?

M：Yes, about two years ago, but this is the first time I have had it checked out.

T：After you're infected with the herpes simplex virus, it <u>remains dormant</u> in your nerves. The virus is reactivated and symptoms begin to appear when your immune system is weakened by a cold, stress, or exposure to strong UV radiation for example.

M：Is there any way to cure it completely?

T：Unfortunately, no. Whenever you have an <u>itchy</u> or <u>tingling sensation</u> on the lips, please come see me as soon as possible. Early use of anti-viral drugs can reduce the symptoms and prevent the spread of the virus.

M：Is it contagious?

T：Yes. You should avoid all <u>physical contact</u> with others until the symptoms disappear. Be especially careful around babies, as the virus can have severe effects for them. The virus can persist for several days, and blisters usually take two to four weeks to heal completely. During this time the virus is highly contagious. Cold sores <u>tend to reappear</u> at the same spot but are usually less severe after the first outbreak. Don't touch the blisters, and be sure to take <u>your medicine on schedule</u>. That will help them heal faster.

M：Okay, doctor. Thanks very much!

 Key words in the dialogue

blister：水疱
tingle：ひりひりする
cold sore：単純疱疹
herpes simplex virus：単純疱疹ウイルス
remain dormant：潜んでいる
symptom：症状，徴候
immune system：免疫システム
itchy：かゆみ
contagious：感染する，伝染する
on schedule：予定通りに，時間通りに

Exercise 4

Let's learn some useful phrases.

Phrases to memorize

1. After you're infected with the herpes simplex virus, it remains dormant in your nerves.
   単純疱疹ウイルスに感染すると，神経内に潜むことになります．

2. Is there any way to cure it completely?
   完治させる方法はありますか．

3. Is it contagious?
   伝染しますか．

4. You should avoid all physical contact with others until the symptoms disappear.
   症状がなくなるまで，ほかの人との接触を避けてください．

5. Don't touch the blisters, and be sure to take your medicine on schedule.
   水疱には触らないでください．薬は定められた時間と回数を守って飲んでください．

Reading 9

Herpes Simplex Virus

There are two types of herpes simplex viruses: herpes simplex virus type 1 (HSV-1) and herpes simplex virus type 2 (HSV-2). Generally, HSV-1 causes oral herpes whereas HSV-2 causes genital herpes. However, both types of viruses can cause both oral and genital diseases. The meaning of the term "herpes" in Greek is to creep or crawl, indicating the spread of blisters (fluid filled swellings) in infections with HSV.

Herpes Simplex Virus type 1 (HSV-1) Infection

HSV-1 is a highly contagious infection, which is common and endemic throughout the world. Most HSV-1 infections are acquired during childhood, and the infection is lifelong. The vast majority of HSV-1 infections are oral herpes (infections in or around the mouth), but a proportion of HSV-1 infections are genital herpes (infections in the genital area).

The natural history of HSV-1 infection can be divided into 3 stages: primary infection, latency, and recurrent infection. Primary infection refers to the initial exposure of an individual who does not have antibodies to the virus. It is usually asymptomatic and the majority of people with HSV-1 infection are unaware they are infected. Once the primary infection is established, the virus enters sensory nerves and is transported to the associated sensory ganglion. Here the virus remains latent and the trigeminal ganglion of the 5th cranial nerve (trigeminal nerve) is the most common site for the virus to remain in a latent state.

Signs and Symptoms

As for symptomatic cases, the affected oral mucosa develops

herpes simplex virus
単純疱疹ウイルス

oral herpes
口腔ヘルペス

genital herpes
性器ヘルペス

creep/crawl　這う

blister　水疱

infection　感染

contagious　伝染性

lifelong　生涯

primary infection
一次感染

latency (latent period)
潜伏期

recurrent infection
再発感染

antibody　抗体

asymptomatic
無症候の

sensory nerve
感覚神経

sensory ganglion
感覚神経節

trigeminal ganglion
三叉神経節

cranial nerve
脳神経

oral mucosa (oral mucous membrane)
口腔粘膜

numerous small vesicles which eventually rupture leading to sore mouth lesions. The onset of these symptomatic cases is sudden and often accompanied by fever and nausea. Ulcers on the lips are commonly referred to as "cold sores." Infected persons will often experience a tingling, itching or burning sensation around their mouth, before the appearance of sores. After initial infection, the blisters or ulcers can periodically recur.

Genital herpes caused by HSV-1 can be asymptomatic or can have mild symptoms that go unrecognized. When symptoms do occur, genital herpes is characterized by 1 or more genital blisters or ulcers. After an initial genital herpes episode, which may be severe, symptoms may recur.

Scope of the Problem

In 2012, an estimated 3.7 billion people under the age of 50, or 67% of the population, had HSV-1 infection. The estimated prevalence of the infection was highest in Africa (87%) and lowest in the Americas (40-50%). With respect to genital HSV-1 infection, 140 million people aged 15-49-years were estimated to have genital HSV-1 infection worldwide in 2012, but prevalence varied substantially by region. Most genital HSV-1 infections are estimated to occur in the Americas, Europe, and Western Pacific, where HSV-1 continues to be acquired well into adulthood. In other regions, for example in Africa, most HSV-1 infections are acquired in childhood, before the age of sexual maturity.

Transmission

HSV-1 is mainly transmitted by oral-to-oral contact to cause oral herpes infection, via contact with the HSV-1 virus in sores, saliva, and surfaces in or around the mouth. However, HSV-1 can also be transmitted to the genital area through oral-genital contact to cause genital herpes. HSV-1 can be transmitted from oral or skin surfaces that appear normal and when there are no symptoms present. However, the greatest risk of transmission is

vesicle　小胞

rupture　破裂する

sore mouth lesions
口内炎

nausea　悪寒, 吐き気

cold sores
口唇ヘルペス

burning sensation
灼熱感

prevalence　有病率

sexual maturity
性的成熟

when there are active sores.

Possible Complications

In immunocompromised people, such as those with advanced HIV infection, HSV-1 can have more severe symptoms and more frequent recurrences. In addition, neonatal herpes can occur when an infant is exposed to HSV in the genital tract during delivery. This is a rare condition but can lead to lasting neurologic disability or death. The risk for neonatal herpes is greatest when a mother acquires HSV infection for the first time in late pregnancy. Furthermore, recurrent symptoms of oral herpes may be uncomfortable and can lead to some social stigma and psychological distress. With genital herpes, these factors can have an important impact on the quality of life and sexual relationships.

Treatment

Antiviral medications, such as Acyclovir, Famciclovir, and Valacyclovir, are the most effective medications available for people infected with HSV. These can help to reduce the severity and frequency of symptoms but cannot cure the infection.

immunocompromised people
免疫不全の人々

HIV infection
HIV感染

neonatal herpes
新生児ヘルペス

genital tract
生殖器

neurologic disability
神経障害

social stigma
社会的不名誉, 汚名

psychological distress
心理的苦痛

Exercise 5

T or F

If the following sentence is true mark T (true), if it is not true mark F (false)

1. ____ Once you get infected with the herpes simplex virus, it lies dormant in the nerves for your entire life.

2. ____ HSV-1 is a low contagious infection.

3. ____ In 2012, an estimated 3.7 million people under the age of 50 had HSV-1 infection.

4. ____ The estimated prevalence of the infection was highest in Asia (87%) and lowest in Africa (40-50%).

5. ____ HSV-1 is mainly transmitted by oral to oral contact to cause infection in and around the mouth (oral herpes).

6. ____ Neonatal herpes can occur when an infant is exposed to HSV in the genital tract during delivery.

7. ____ Antiviral medications such as Acyclovir can cure HSV infection.

8. ____ In immunocompromised people, such as those with advanced HIV infection, HSV-1 can have mild symptoms and no recurrences.

References : Oral and Maxillofacial Pathology (Fourth Edition) By Brad W. Neville, Douglas D. Damm, Carl M. Allen, Angela C. Chi
WHO (World Health Organization) website on Herpes simplex virus (https://www.who.int/news-room/fact-sheets/detail/herpes-simplex-virus)

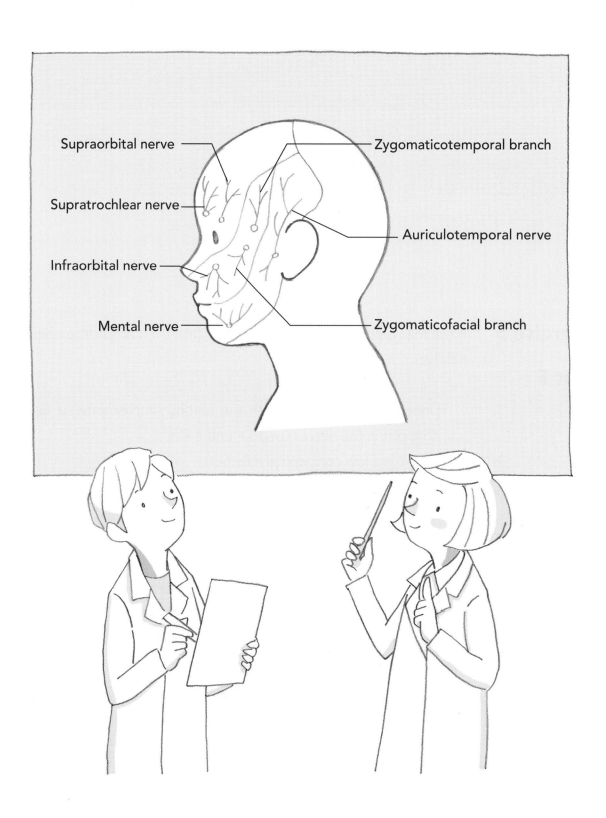

10 The Temporomandibular Joint

Dental Interview

Exercise 1 Listen to the dialogue and answer the following questions.

Interview questions

1. Why is Mr. Schmidt visiting a dental university?

   _____

2. What kind of symptoms does he have?

   _____

3. Where exactly is the pain?

   _____

4. What is the TMJ?

   _____

5. How many treatments does the dentist talk about?

   _____

6. What is the dentist's recommendation?

   _____

Listen to the dialogue and fill in the missing words.

Fill in the blanks

> H : Ms. Hayashi, a receptionist
>
> S : Mr. Schmidt, a 50-year-old carpenter
>
> K : Dr. Kato, a dentist

At a dental university

H : Good morning. Can I help you?

S : Good morning. My name is Ben Schmidt. I've been having some _____ _____. I'm already a patient at this university.

H : OK! Can you spell your name for me?

S : It's Ben, B-E-N...Schmidt, S-C-H-M-I-D-T.

H : All right. Give me a second. Well, here's your name. We have a TMD center on the third floor of this hospital. TMD stands for temporomandibular disorder.

At the TMD Center

K : Hello Mr. Schmidt! My name is Dr. Kato. I'll be treating you. So what brings you here today?

S : Well, I have been having really bad jaw pain, and can't open my mouth wide. Also, my jaw _____ when I open my mouth.

K : I see. How's your general health? Have you had any _____, _____, headaches or other medical problems?

S : No, I haven't. I'm absolutely fine.

K : OK, you can lie back in the dental chair and relax. Can you open your mouth? Where do you have the pain?

S : Well, I have had bad pain near my ear.

K : And when does it hurt?

S : It hurts almost every day, and has lasted about a year.

K : Is the pain here, in the jaw, or this joint? We call it the _____ _____, or TMJ for short. Or is it in the muscles?

S：Yes, it's in that joint.

K：OK, let me take a look. Can you open your mouth again? I'm going to take an X-ray.

After the treatment

K：OK, the treatment's finished. I can recommend two things for you. First, you need to exercise your jaw. Try exercising it for five minutes, three times a day, after each meal. This will help with opening your jaw. Second, you need to change your eating habits. Eat more soft foods and avoid chewing gum.

S：I understand. OK, I'll try the exercises and change my eating habits.

K：Good. Take care of yourself.

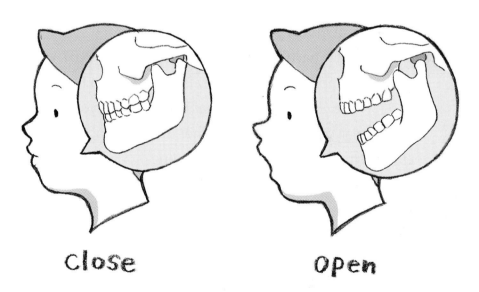

close   open

Exercise 3

Read the dialogue and check the answers.

Learn the points

> H : Ms. Hayashi, a receptionist
>
> S : Mr. Schmidt, a 50-year-old carpenter
>
> K : Dr. Kato, a dentist

At a dental university

H : Good morning. Can I help you?

S : Good morning. My name is Ben Schmidt. I've been having some jaw pain. I'm already a patient at this university.

H : OK! Can you spell your name for me?

S : It's Ben, B-E-N...Schmidt, S-C-H-M-I-D-T.

H : All right. Give me a second. Well, here's your name. We have a TMD center on the third floor of this hospital. TMD stands for temporomandibular disorder.

At the TMD Center

K : Hello Mr. Schmidt! My name is Dr. Kato. I'll be treating you. So what brings you here today?

S : Well, I have been having really bad jaw pain, and can't open my mouth wide. Also, my jaw clicks when I open my mouth.

K : I see. How's your general health? Have you had any arthritis, dialysis, headaches or other medical problems?

S : No, I haven't. I'm absolutely fine.

K : OK, you can lie back in the dental chair and relax. Can you open your mouth? Where do you have the pain?

S : Well, I have had bad pain near my ear.

K : And when does it hurt?

S : It hurts almost every day, and has lasted about a year.

K : Is the pain here, in the jaw, or this joint? We call it the temporomandibular joint, or TMJ for short. Or is it in the muscles?

S：Yes, it's in that joint.

K：OK, let me take a look. Can you open your mouth again? I'm going to take an X-ray.

After the treatment

K：OK, the treatment's finished. I can recommend two things for you. First, you need to exercise your jaw. Try exercising it for five minutes, three times a day, after each meal. This will help with opening your jaw. Second, you need to change your eating habits. Eat more soft foods and avoid chewing gum.

S：I understand. OK, I'll try the exercises and change my eating habits.

K：Good. Take care of yourself.

 Key words in the dialogue

jaw pain：顎の痛み
arthritis：関節炎
dialysis：透析
temporomandibular joint（TMJ）：顎関節

Exercise 4

Phrases to memorize

Let's learn some useful phrases.

1. **Can you spell your name for me?**
   お名前の綴りを教えてください.

2. **Where do you have the pain?**
   どこが痛みますか.

3. **When does it hurt?**
   いつ痛みますか.

Reading 10

The Temporomandibular Joint (TMJ)

The temporomandibular joint (TMJ) is actually two joints—one on each side of the jawbone—that connect the jawbone to the skull. The word temporomandibular refers to the temporal bone of the skull, and the mandible, or lower jawbone. While joints such as the elbow or knee joints function independently, the two sides of the TMJ form a bilateral joint that operates as a single unit. Whenever you open or close your mouth, the two sides of the TMJ move together.

Dislocation of the TMJ can occur due to various reasons. Simply yawning or taking a large bite can lead to anterior (forward) dislocation of the TMJ, in which the heads of the mandible pass anteriorly to the articular tubercles. In this case the mandible remains wide open and cannot be closed. Dislocation of the TMJ can also occur during tooth extraction if excessive force is placed on the mandible. In other cases, a dislocated TMJ may result from a blow to the chin while the mouth is open, for example in a physical assault, sports injury, traffic accident, accident at home, or workplace accident. Dislocations may be bilateral (affecting both sides) or unilateral (affecting only one side), although bilateral dislocations are more common. If caused by an accident or assault, then dislocation may occur together with fracture of the mandible. Superior (upward) dislocation and posterior (backward) dislocation of the TMJ are very rare, and usually the result of severe trauma.

Signs of a dislocated jaw may include pain, poor alignment of the upper and lower teeth, and difficulty speaking. You might also notice the upper or lower jaw protruding too far, resulting in an

temporomandibular joint (TMJ)	顎関節
skull	頭蓋骨
temporal bone	側頭骨
mandible	下顎
bilateral	両側の
dislocation	脱臼
anterior	前方の
articular tubercle	関節結節
unilateral	片側の
fracture	骨折
superior	上方の
posterior	後方の
trauma	外傷
alignment (of teeth)	歯並び
protruding	前突する

overbite or underbite.

 Dislocation of the TMJ will likely be treated as a medical emergency requiring urgent treatment by a doctor or dentist. Sometimes the jaw can be manipulated back into the correct position by hand, under local anaesthetic. However, in certain cases surgery is necessary. During surgery on the TMJ, care must be taken to preserve the surrounding nerves.

overbite　過蓋咬合

underbite　反対咬合

manipulate
動かす, 操作する

local anaesthetic
局所麻酔

Exercise 5

T or F

If the following sentence is true mark T (true), if it is not true mark F (false).

1. ☐ The two sides of the TMJ function independently of each other.
2. ☐ Dislocation of the TMJ has many different causes.
3. ☐ Dislocation usually occurs on both sides of the mandible.
4. ☐ Dislocation and fracture of the mandible sometimes occur together.
5. ☐ Replacing a dislocated TMJ is a simple procedure that anyone can do.

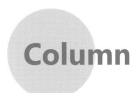

Column

Talking to patients—Tips for successful communication

Look at the dialogue and ask yourself: Why does the patient find it difficult to answer?

> Dentist : So, you have a pain in your mandible?
> Patient : In my...sorry?
> Dentist : Your mandible...your lower jaw.
> Patient : Oh, yes.
> Dentist : Where exactly does it hurt? Please tell me. Is it the temporomandibular joint?
> Patient : Uh...here.
> Dentist : The left TMJ. I see. When did it start, and how would you describe the pain?
> Patient : Umm, I'm not sure...and I don't really know how to explain it.

There are several reasons why this patient couldn't answer smoothly.

1) Most patients do not know much technical vocabulary.

Terms like *mandible* and *TMJ* are basic vocabulary for dentists, but many first-time patients won't understand them. A question like "So, you have a pain in your mandible?" will be confusing if your patient doesn't know what the *mandible* is. As a general rule, don't use technical vocabulary without explaining its meaning, or use simpler terms if possible. In the case of the maxilla and mandible, you can just say *upper jaw* and *lower jaw*. For the TMJ, you could just point and say, "This joint here?"

2) Showing is often easier than telling.

Rather than *telling* you exactly where they have pain, patients often find it easier to *show* you where they have pain, and so often point and say something like "around this bone" or "this tooth here." You can encourage this by asking patients "Can you show me where the pain is?" or "Where does it hurt? Can you point to it?"

3) Patients may not remember exactly when their symptoms started.

Especially if the onset was gradual, a patient may be unable to say exactly when their symptoms started. If it was 11 days ago, the patient might only remember this as "more than a week ago" or "about 2 weeks ago." The longer the elapsed time, the vaguer the patient's memory is likely to be (Was it 3 months ago? Or 6 months?). If a patient seems unsure, you can help them by making suggestions ("More than 2 weeks?", "Less than a month?").

4) Many patients struggle to describe pain in words.

Suffering pain is (hopefully) a rare thing for most people, and not something they usually need to describe in words. "How would you describe the pain?" may be a difficult question to answer. Again, you can help your patients by offering suggestions, such as "How would you describe the pain? Is it a sharp, stabbing pain, or more of a dull, throbbing pain?" or "On a scale of 1 to 10, with 10 being the worst pain you know, how would you rate this pain?"

Summary
 · Avoid technical vocabulary.
 · When you have to use technical vocabulary, explain its meaning.
 · Where necessary, allow patients to show you rather than tell you.
 · Suggest words and phrases to help patients answer your questions.

Challenge!! In the dialogue on page 94, how would you talk to the patient if you were the dentist? Rewrite the dialogue using more suitable questions.

Challenge!!

Sialolithiasis

Dental Interview

Exercise 1   Listen to the dialogue and answer the following questions.

Interview questions

1. Why did Mr. Scheinin decide to visit to his home dentist?

   _____

2. Does he have any pain?

   _____

3. When do his symptoms come?

   _____

4. What kind examination has Dr. Hamura done?

   _____

5. Which department will the referral letter go to?

   _____

Exercise 2

Fill in the blanks

Listen to the dialogue and complete the following sentences.

> S ：Mr. Scheinin, a 38-years-old male came from Finland and is now living in Japan
>
> H ：Dr. Hamura, home dentist of Mr. Scheinin

Mr. Scheinin has received his oral health check-up annually in his home dental clinic. This time, he had an emergency visit to his dentist because of some problems with his oral health.

S ：Good afternoon, Dr. Hamura.

H ：Good afternoon, Mr. Scheinin. What _____ _____ here today? You had an annual oral health check-up nine months ago, didn't you?

S ：Yes I did Dr. Hamura. I did not have any problems with my teeth that time. But I have become recently _____ _____ my oral health.

H ：You have become anxious about your mouth, have you?

S ：It is not the inside of my mouth, but under the lower jaw. I have had a swelling under the right side of my lower jaw.

H ：Is it still swollen?

S ：No, it isn't. When I eat, it becomes swollen.

H ：Is it swollen whenever you eat?

S ：It _____ ____ ____ _____, but lately it swells with every meal. The swelling disappears in about 30 minutes.

H ：Are the symptoms painful?

S ：No, I don't have pain. When I press the swollen area, something like saliva comes out of my mouth.

H ：I see. Then let me touch your mouth and jaw.

<Bimanual palpation (examination) of submandibular salivary gland is done.>

H ：I can feel something small and hard. I think it is a salivary stone, so let's _____ ___ _____ for confirmation.

S ： Dr. Hamura, is it something bad?

H ： I don't think so. The salivary duct which saliva comes out of seems to be blocked and clogged. It is a disease called sialolithiasis. Although it is not malignant, it is better to be treated by a maxillofacial surgeon. I _____ _____ _____ _____ the department of oral and maxillofacial surgery at a university hospital, so please take my referral letter and the data of the radiograph to be taken.

S ： Thank you, Dr. Hamura. I will go to the university hospital as soon as possible.

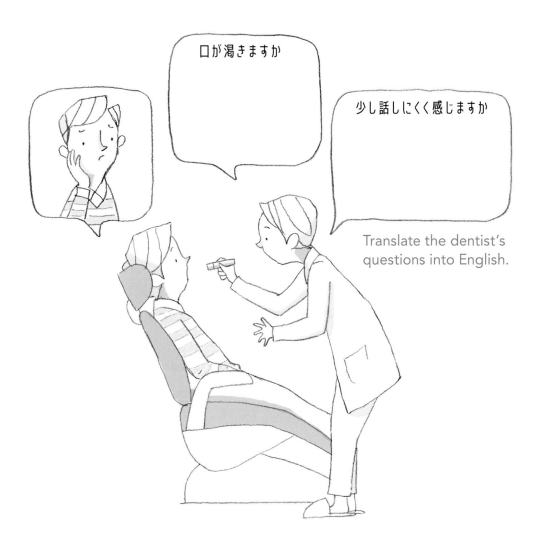

Translate the dentist's questions into English.

11 Sialolithiasis

Exercise 3

Read the dialogue and check the answers.

Learn the points

> S ： Mr. Scheinin, a 38-years-old male came from Finland and is now living in Japan
>
> H ： Dr. Hamura, home dentist of Mr. Scheinin

Mr. Scheinin has received his oral health check-up annually in his home dental clinic. This time, he had an emergency visit to his dentist because of some problems with his oral health.

S ： Good afternoon, Dr. Hamura.

H ： Good afternoon, Mr. Scheinin. What <u>brought you</u> here today? You had an annual oral health check-up nine months ago, didn't you?

S ： Yes I did Dr. Hamura. I did not have any problems with my teeth that time. But I have become recently <u>anxious about</u> my oral health.

H ： You have become anxious about your mouth, have you?

S ： It is not the inside of my mouth, but under the lower jaw. I have had a swelling under the right side of my lower jaw.

H ： Is it still swollen?

S ： No, it isn't. When I eat, it becomes swollen.

H ： Is it swollen whenever you eat?

S ： It <u>used to be occasionally</u>, but lately it swells with every meal. The swelling disappears in about 30 minutes.

H ： Are the symptoms painful?

S ： No, I don't have pain. When I press the swollen area, something like saliva comes out of my mouth.

H ： I see. Then let me touch your mouth and jaw.

<Bimanual palpation (examination) of submandibular salivary gland is done.>

H ： I can feel something small and hard. I think it is a salivary stone, so let's <u>take a radiograph</u> for confirmation.

S ：Dr. Hamura, is it something bad?

H ：I don't think so. The salivary duct which saliva comes out of seems to be blocked and clogged. It is a disease called sialolithiasis. Although it is not malignant, it is better to be treated by a maxillofacial surgeon. I <u>will refer you to</u> the department of oral and maxillofacial surgery at a university hospital, so please take my referral letter and the data of the radiograph to be taken.

S ：Thank you, Dr. Hamura. I will go to the university hospital as soon as possible.

 Key words in the dialogue

sialolithiasis：唾石症
oral health check-up：口腔健康診査
　regular oral health check-up：定期的な口腔健康診査
　an annual oral health check-up：年に1度の定期健診
　biannual oral health check-up：年に2度の定期健診
become anxious about：〜が気になる
palpation：触診（指や手で患者さんの体を直接触って診断する方法）
bimanual palpation：双手診（両手を使った触診）
saliva：唾液
salivary stone：唾石
malignant：悪性の
take a radiograph / take an X-ray：エックス線写真を撮る
　radiograph / X-ray photograph / roentgenograph / rentgenogram：エックス線写真
refer you to department of maxillofacial surgery：口腔外科を紹介する
referral letter：紹介状

◆Let's look at the images of salivary stone

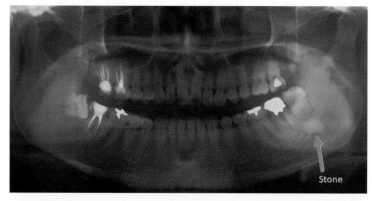

Salivary stone on panoramic tomography X-ray

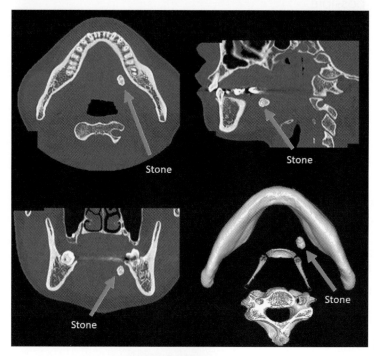

Salivary stone on CT image

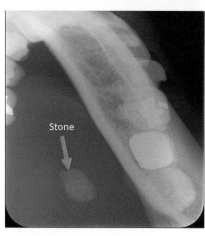

Salivary stone on occlusal radiography of mandible
（写真：3枚とも日本歯科大学附属病院放射線診断科より提供）

Exercise 4   Let's learn some useful phrases.

Phrases to memorize

1. Are the symptoms painful?
   痛みはありますか.

2. Let me touch your mouth and jaw.
   口と顎を触ります.

3. I will refer you to the department of oral and maxillofacial surgery at a university hospital.
   大学病院の口腔顎顔面外科に紹介します.
   医療連携で紹介する場合には，introduce ではなく refer を用います.
   同様に，他院への紹介状も letter of introduction ではなく，referral letter を用います.

Reading 11

Sialolithiasis

Definition

Sialolithiasis is defined as disease where salivary stones, or calculi, develop in salivary glands or ducts, and usually presents with sialadenitis. It frequently occurs in adult males and smokers. Salivary stones are mostly found in the submandibular glands and less often in parotid, sublingual, and minor salivary glands. They usually develop unilaterally, but rarely bilaterally. Salivary stones are formed by the deposition of salivary calcium carbonate on microstructures (for example, foreign substances or microorganisms that have entered the salivary glands or ducts, and desquamated epithelium etc.) present in the salivary glands or ducts.

Salivary Stone

A salivary stone is small at first but gradually grows larger and comes in various shapes and hardness. Rough surfaces and sharp edges of the stone can damage the contacting epithelium and cause inflammation. Chronic inflammation might lead to sialadenitis. Large salivary stones can inhibit the discharge saliva from the salivary gland. Clinically, this results in xerostomia, local swelling and pain.

Symptoms

The main clinical symptoms of sialolithiasis are swelling, spontaneous pain and/or tenderness in the salivary glands during meals. The pain caused by blockages of saliva from the salivary gland is called salivary colic. Symptoms are often asymptomatic and may be accidently found on diagnostic imaging performed for other purposes such as annual oral health check-up.

sialolithiasis　唾石症

salivary stone　唾石

calculi　結石

salivary gland
唾液腺

salivary duct
唾液管

sialadenitis
唾液腺炎

submandibular glands
顎下腺

parotid　耳下腺

sublingual　舌下

desquamated
はがれた, 落屑した

epithelium　上皮

chronic　慢性的な

xerostomia
口腔乾燥症

spontaneous pain
自発痛

salivary colic
唾疝痛

asymptomatic
無症候性の

Diagnosis

Diagnosis of sialolithiasis is based on clinical symptoms, visual inspection, and palpation. If large salivary stones are located close to the salivary gland orifice, the salivary stones may be visible in the oral cavity. Even relatively small salivary stones can be confirmed by palpation if they are in the salivary gland ducts. A definite diagnosis is made with X-rays or CT images.

palpation 触診

orifice 開口部

Treatment

For asymptomatic or small-sized salivary stones, the first option for treatment is follow-up after anti-inflammatory therapy because spontaneous excretion of salivary stones is expected. Treatment may involve surgery to remove salivary stones in patients who cannot expect spontaneous discharge. The stones in salivary gland orifices or ducts, are removed by an intraoral surgery. If there is atrophy of the salivary gland, repeated inflammation or impaired function of the salivary gland, the salivary stones are removed together with the salivary gland. A method of removing salivary stones by inserting a fine endoscope through a duct orifice can also be performed.

spontaneous excretion
自然排出

atrophy 萎縮

impaired function
機能障害

endoscope 内視鏡

Exercise 5

T or F

If the following sentence is true mark T (true), if it is not true mark F (false).

1. _____ Salivary stones usually develop bilateral.
2. _____ Calcium is the main component of salivary stone.
3. _____ The surface of salivary stones is smooth and the shape is round.
4. _____ Palpation is suitable examination for diagnose salivary stone.
5. _____ Since salivary stones have radiolucency, they appear white in X-rays.

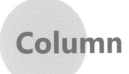

Column

専門用語の成り立ち

　からだの組織や病名を表す英語の学術・専門用語は，ギリシャ語をもとにつくられている言葉が多くあります．そのため，学術・専門用語がどのようにして成り立っているかを理解すると，言葉を覚えるのに役立ちます．唾石症に関係する学術・専門用語も例外ではありません．

　唾石の英語は，患者さんなどに説明するときには "salivary stone" もしくは "salivary calculus" を使います．"sialolith" は，唾石を意味する学術・専門用語ですので，医療関係者はこちらの言葉も覚えなければなりません．接頭語の "sial" もしくは "sialo" は，唾液を意味します．"sialo" に続く "lith" は石・結石・石灰化を意味する連結形ですので，"sialo+lith" で唾石となります．

　唾石症は "sialolithiasis" です．接尾語の "iasis" は病名や病状を表しますので，唾石を意味する "sialolith" に病名の "iasis" をくっつけて "sialolith+iasis" 唾石症となります．

　唾液腺炎は "sialadenitis" です．唾液の "sial" に，腺を意味する "aden" がくっつくと唾液腺 "sialaden" となり，炎症を意味する接尾語 "itis" が最後尾に加わると唾液腺炎 "sial+aden+itis" になります．

　唾液管閉塞 "sialostenosis" は唾液の "sialo" に狭窄症を意味する "stenosis" が組み合わさっています．狭窄症とは体内の管状組織が異常に狭まる症状です．"osis" は症状を表す接尾語です．

参考文献 (Reading)：榎本昭二ほか監修：最新口腔外科学 第 5 版，医歯薬出版，2017
中原 泉ほか編：常用歯科辞典 第 4 版，医歯薬出版，2016
Marchal F., Dulguerov P.,：Sialolithiasis Management The state of the Art, *Arch Otolaryngol Head Neck Surg.* 2003;129(9):951-956
(https://jamanetwork.com/journals/jamaotolaryngology/fullarticle/483947)
参考文献 (Column)：菅原美佳：医学英語の語彙力の教科を目指す効果的な教育方法についての考察，東北医科薬科大学教養教育関係論文集 31 号 1-14, 2017
MEDO 医学英語語幹－医歯薬英語辞書

12 Inferior Alveolar Nerve Block

Dental Interview

Exercise 1   Listen to the dialogue and answer the following questions.

Interview questions

1. Why is Mr. Smith visiting a dental clinic?

   _____

2. How does he describe the pain?

   _____

3. What kind of treatments is Dr. Yamada performing?

   _____

4. What is a panoramic X-ray?

   _____

5. What is the dentist's recommendation?

   _____

Listen to the dialogue and complete the following sentences.

> S : Mr. Smith, a 45-year-old school teacher
>
> Y : Dr. Yamada, a dentist

Around 2 pm at a dental clinic

Y : Good afternoon Mr. Smith. What brings you here today?

S : Hello doctor. I have a toothache.

Y : Which tooth is it?

S : It's in the back, in my right lower jaw.

Y : All right. I'll take a look at that tooth and your other teeth and gums. This is a percussion test. Are you still in pain? Do you feel any pain in the tooth?

S : Ouch! That tooth really hurts.

Y : Can you describe the pain? Is it _____, _____, or numbing pain? And how long have you had it?

S : It's a throbbing pain. I have had it for about two days.

Y : I'd like to take a panoramic X-ray.

S : What's that?

Y : It's a _____ scan of the upper and lower _____. It produces an image of all your teeth in two dimensions. I can take a look at the tooth that's bothering you, along with all your other teeth. I'll let you know if I find any other problems.

After X-ray inspection

Y : Mr. Smith, the panoramic X-ray shows a _____ tooth in your right lower jaw. It's your wisdom tooth, the right lower third molar! I recommend that you have it taken out; otherwise the _____ _____ will spread to the neighbouring tooth. You don't appear to have any other problems with your other teeth. The hygienist will examine your gums later.

S : Doctor, are there any alternatives to having it pulled? I'm really worried about having it taken out.

Y：Well, it would be better to take it out. Here, take a look at the X-ray. You see, the tooth is not only decayed, it's also partially _____. If you have it extracted, your bite won't change. And it's in a bad condition. It's not a good idea to leave it. If you have no treatments, the tooth will probably have further tooth decay.

S：OK. I understand.

Y：All right. I'm going to inject some anaesthesia. I will give an inferior alveolar nerve block. First, I'm going to use a little topical anaesthesia. Then I'm going to inject the local _____. Have you ever had an allergic reaction to anaesthesia?

S：No, I'm not allergic to any medicines.

Y：OK. If you feel any pain, please raise your hand.

S：All right.

After anaesthetic injection

Y：Please rinse your mouth. How is it?

S：My tooth is getting _____.

Y：OK, let's wait about 5 more minutes.

5 minutes later

Y：Mr. Smith. Do your gums feel numb?

S：Yes, definitely.

Y：Well, I'm going to take out the tooth now. If you feel any pain, raise your hand.

S：OK. I understand.

Exercise 3 Read the dialogue and check the answers.

Learn the points

> S ： Mr. Smith, a 45-year-old school teacher
>
> Y ： Dr. Yamada, a dentist

Around 2 pm at a dental clinic

Y ： Good afternoon Mr. Smith. What brings you here today?

S ： Hello doctor. I have a toothache.

Y ： Which tooth is it?

S ： It's in the back, in my right lower jaw.

Y ： All right. I'll take a look at that tooth and your other teeth and gums. This is a percussion test. Are you still in pain? Do you feel any pain in the tooth?

S ： Ouch! That tooth really hurts.

Y ： Can you describe the pain? Is it <u>throbbing, pulsating</u>, or numbing pain? And how long have you had it?

S ： It's a throbbing pain. I have had it for about two days.

Y ： I'd like to take a panoramic X-ray.

S ： What's that?

Y ： It's a <u>panoramic</u> scan of the upper and lower <u>jaws</u>. It produces an image of all your teeth in two dimensions. I can take a look at the tooth that's bothering you, along with all your other teeth. I'll let you know if I find any other problems.

After X-ray inspection

Y ： Mr. Smith, the panoramic X-ray shows a <u>decayed</u> tooth in your right lower jaw. It's your wisdom tooth, the right lower third molar! I recommend that you have it taken out; otherwise the <u>tooth decay</u> will spread to the neighbouring tooth. You don't appear to have any other problems with your other teeth. The hygienist will examine your gums later.

S ： Doctor, are there any alternatives to having it pulled? I'm really worried about having it taken out.

Y：Well, it would be better to take it out. Here, take a look at the X-ray. You see, the tooth is not only decayed, it's also partially <u>embedded</u>. If you have it extracted, your bite won't change. And it's in a bad condition. It's not a good idea to leave it. If you have no treatments, the tooth will probably have further tooth decay.

S：OK. I understand.

Y：All right. I'm going to inject some anaesthesia. I will give an inferior alveolar nerve block. First, I'm going to use a little topical anaesthesia. Then I'm going to inject the local <u>anaesthesia</u>. Have you ever had an allergic reaction to anaesthesia?

S：No, I'm not allergic to any medicines.

Y：OK. If you feel any pain, please raise your hand.

S：All right.

After anaesthetic injection

Y：Please rinse your mouth. How is it?

S：My tooth is getting <u>numb</u>.

Y：OK, let's wait about 5 more minutes.

5 minutes later

Y：Mr. Smith. Do your gums feel numb?

S：Yes, definitely.

Y：Well, I'm going to take out the tooth now. If you feel any pain, raise your hand.

S：OK. I understand.

Key words in the dialogue

percussion test：打診
throbbing pain：ずきずきする痛み
pulsating pain：拍動痛
numbing pain：感覚がなくなるような痛み
panoramic X-ray：パノラマエックス線
decayed tooth / dental caries：むし歯
numb：麻痺している
take out / pull out / extract：抜歯する
anaesthesia：麻酔
　topical anaesthesia：表面麻酔
　local anaesthesia：局所麻酔
inferior alveolar nerve block：下歯槽神経ブロック

Exercise 4

Let's learn some useful phrases.

Phrases to memorize

1. Are you still in pain?
   今も痛みますか.

2. Can you describe the pain?
   痛みを説明してくださいますか.

3. Have you ever had an allergic reaction to anaesthesia?
   今までに麻酔のアレルギー反応がでたことがありますか.

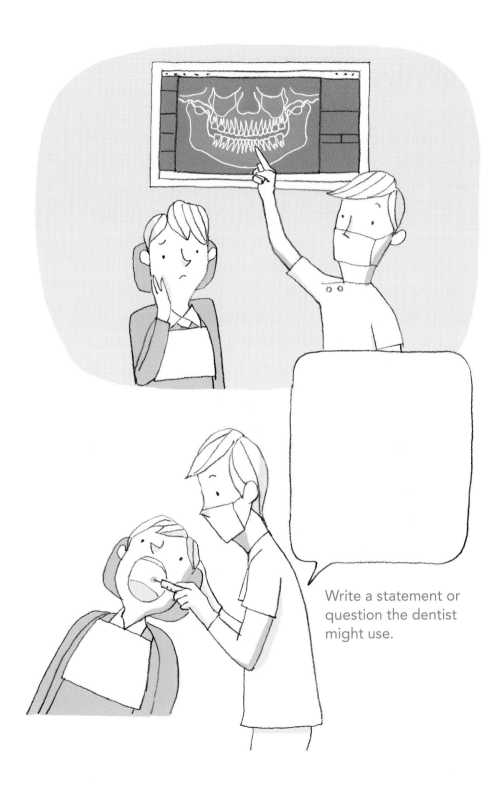

Write a statement or question the dentist might use.

12 Inferior Alveolar Nerve Block

Reading 12

Inferior Alveolar Nerve Block

The inferior alveolar nerve block is the most common injection technique used in dentistry and performed regularly in dental clinics. The inferior alveolar nerve is anaesthetized by injecting the anaesthetic fluid around the mandibular region. When an inferior alveolar nerve block is successful, all the lower teeth are anaesthetized to the midline. The skin and mucous membrane of the lower lip, the labial alveolar mucosa and gingiva, and the skin of the chin are also anaesthetized because they are supplied by the mental nerve, the terminal branch of the inferior alveolar nerve. Knowledge of anatomy in the inferior alveolar nerve is especially important to perform the procedure.

Basic Anatomy of the Mandibular Nerve

The 3rd branch of the trigeminal nerve, the mandibular nerve exits the skull through the foramen ovale and then divides into the anterior and posterior divisions with the main nerve trunk below the foramen. The main trunk of the mandibular nerve gives two branches, namely a) the nerve to medial pterygoid muscle and b) a meningeal branch which goes back to the cranium through the foramen spinosum; this branch runs superiorly through the foramen spinosum to supply the dura mater of the middle cranial fossa. Inferior to the two branches, the main trunk splits into an anterior and a posterior trunk.

The anterior trunk has the buccal nerve and mainly motor branches that supplies the masseter, temporal, lateral pterygoid muscles. The posterior trunk has the inferior alveolar nerve, the lingual nerve, the auriculotemporal nerve that gives sensory

inferior alveolar
nerve block
下歯槽神経ブロック

mucous membrane
粘膜

labial alveolar mucosa
唇側歯槽粘膜

mental nerve
オトガイ神経

mandibular nerve
下顎神経

trigeminal nerve
三叉神経

foramen ovale
卵円孔

medial pterygoid
muscle
内側翼突筋

meningeal branch
硬膜枝

foramen spinosum
棘孔

middle cranial fossa
中頭蓋窩

buccal nerve　頬神経

masseter muscle
咬筋

temporal muscle
側頭筋

lateral pterygoid
muscle
外側翼突筋

lingual nerve　舌神経

perception to the side of the head and scalp and sends small branches to the external auditory meatus, the tympanic membrane, and the temporomandibular joint.

Basic Anatomy of the Inferior Alveolar Nerve

The inferior alveolar nerve enters the mandibular foramen in the ramus of the mandible and runs below the teeth as far as the mental foramen. The inferior alveolar nerve gives off the mylohyoid nerve, branches to the molar and premolar teeth of the mandibular and the incisive and the mental nerves. The mylohyoid nerve is derived from the inferior alveolar nerve just before the latter enters the mandibular foramen. The mylohyoid nerve sends a branch to the mylohyoid muscle and the anterior belly of the digastric muscle. The branches to the molar and premolar teeth supply the adjoining gingiva. The incisive nerves supply the incisor teeth and form an elaborate plexus. The mental nerve emerges at the mental foramen, and divides into three branches; one branch descends to the skin of the chin, and two branches ascend to the skin and mucous membrane of the lower lip. These three branches communicate with the mandibular branch of the facial nerve.

The Conventional Inferior Alveolar Nerve Block

The inferior alveolar nerve block is the most common technique used in dentistry. Despite its importance, it is associated with a failure rate of 15-20% a figure which represents the highest percentage of all clinical failures achieved using local anaesthesia. The conventional method of blocking the inferior alveolar nerve involves the insertion of the dental needle near the area of the mandibular foramen, where the inferior alveolar nerve is located before it enters the foramen. Some important landmarks need to be recognized by the operator in order to reduce the percentage of failure following the use of this technique. Radiographs are usually available for most patients before treatment and many dentists concentrate on problems related to the dentition and jaw

auriculotemporal nerve
耳介側頭神経

sensory perception
知覚

external auditory meatus
外耳道

tympanic membrane
鼓膜

mylohyoid nerve
顎舌骨神経

mylohyoid muscle
顎舌骨筋

digastric muscle
顎二腹筋

ascend to　上行する

local anaesthesia
局所麻酔

mandibular foramen
下顎孔

dentition　歯列

as seen in these radiographs, but may not use them to estimate the location of the mandibular foramen and other bony landmarks used in the inferior alveolar nerve block. Many studies have shown that the mandibular foramen can easily be located on orthopantomogram (OPG) radiographs.

Exercise 5

T or F

If the following sentence is true mark T (true), if it is not true mark F (false).

1. ☐ The buccal nerve is the branch of the maxillary nerve.
2. ☐ The mandibular nerve has not only motor, but sensory fibers.
3. ☐ The masseter muscle is innervated by the mandibular nerve.
4. ☐ The posterior belly of the digastric muscle is innervated by the mandibular nerve.
5. ☐ The first branch from the mandibular nerve is the meningeal branch, which supply the meninges.

Sources : Anesth Essays Res. 2014, Jan-Apr; 8(1): 3-8 Hesham Khalil

13 Trigeminal Neuralgia

Dental Interview

Exercise 1   Listen to the dialogue and answer the following questions.

Interview questions

1. Why is Ms. Writer visiting a doctor?

   _____

2. Where exactly is the pain?

   _____

3. How does she describe the pain?

   _____

4. What is trigeminal neuralgia?

   _____

5. What is the trigeminal nerve?

   _____

6. What kind of doctor is treating the patient?

   _____

Exercise 2

Listen to the dialogue and complete the following sentences.

Fill in the blanks

W : Ms. Writer, a 50-year-old chief manager at ABC Company

H : Dr. Honda, an oral surgeon

At a dental university

The phone is ringing at 9:00 AM

H : Hello! This is Dr. Honda speaking. May I help you?

W : Hello, doctor. I hope you can help. I have severe pain in my face.

H : Can you describe where it is located exactly?

W : I have pain in my left cheek.

H : All right. Can you come to our university now?

W : Yes I can.

40 minutes later

H : Hello Ms. Writer! I'm Dr. Honda and I spoke to you on the phone earlier. I'll be _____ you today. What can we do for you?

W : I've been _____ from this severe pain. It's a stabbing pain, lasting 15 to 20 seconds, occurring several times a day and it's been so severe that I've even contemplated suicide. The pain seems to be _____ by chewing and by cold wind blowing on my upper lip.

H : Is there anything more you would like to say about your problem?

W : I have the pain in my upper left lip, left cheek, and below my left eye. The pain also _____ _____ my lower eyelid, side of my nose, and the inside of my mouth.

H : Ms. Writer, it's likely that you have trigeminal neuralgia.

W : Trigeminal neuralgia? What's that?

H : Trigeminal neuralgia is a chronic pain condition that affects the 5th _____ _____ which carries sensation from your face to the brain. If you have trigeminal neuralgia, even mild stimulation of the face may trigger jolts of severe pain. A variety of triggers may set off the pain of trigeminal neuralgia, including washing your face, _____ your teeth, and encountering a breeze.

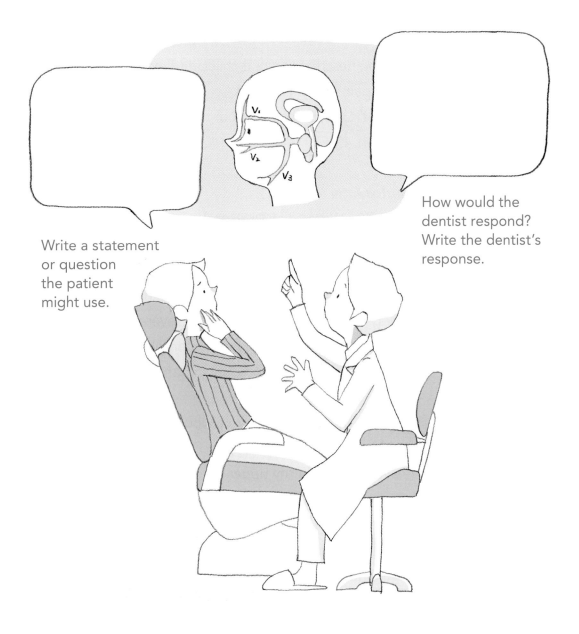

Write a statement or question the patient might use.

How would the dentist respond? Write the dentist's response.

13 Trigeminal Neuralgia

Exercise 3

Read the dialogue and check the answers.

Learn the points

> W : Ms. Writer, a 50-year-old chief manager at ABC Company
>
> H : Dr. Honda, an oral surgeon

At a dental university

The phone is ringing at 9:00 AM

H : Hello! This is Dr. Honda speaking. May I help you?

W : Hello, doctor. I hope you can help. I have severe pain in my face.

H : Can you describe where it is located exactly?

W : I have pain in my left cheek.

H : All right. Can you come to our university now?

W : Yes I can.

40 minutes later

H : Hello Ms. Writer! I'm Dr. Honda and I spoke to you on the phone earlier. I'll be <u>treating</u> you today. What can we do for you?

W : I've been <u>suffering</u> from this severe pain. It's a stabbing pain, lasting 15 to 20 seconds, occurring several times a day and it's been so severe that I've even contemplated suicide. The pain seems to be <u>triggered</u> by chewing and by cold wind blowing on my upper lip.

H : Is there anything more you would like to say about your problem?

W : I have the pain in my upper left lip, left cheek, and below my left eye. The pain also <u>spread to</u> my lower eyelid, side of my nose, and the inside of my mouth.

H : Ms. Writer, it's likely that you have trigeminal neuralgia.

W : Trigeminal neuralgia? What's that?

H : Trigeminal neuralgia is a chronic pain condition that affects the 5th <u>cranial nerve</u> which carries sensation from your face to the brain. If you have trigeminal neuralgia, even mild stimulation of your face may trigger jolts of severe pain. A variety of triggers may set off the pain of trigeminal neuralgia, including washing your face, <u>brushing</u> your teeth, and encountering a breeze.

 Key words in the dialogue

stabbing pain：刺すような痛み
contemplated suicide：計画自殺
trigger：引き起こす，引き金
trigeminal neuralgia / tic douloureux：三叉神経痛
chronic pain：慢性的な痛み
cranial nerve：脳神経
stimulation：刺激
jolts：ショック，衝撃

Exercise 4　Let's learn some useful phrases.

Phrases to memorize

1. Can you describe where it is located exactly?
   痛みの場所を正確に（はっきりと）言えますか.

2. I'll be treating you today.
   本日，担当するのは私です.

3. Is there anything more you would like to say about your problem?
   痛みについてもっと教えていただけますか.

Reading 13

Trigeminal Neuralgia

Description

Trigeminal Neuralgia (trigem-i-nal new-ral-gia), TN, also known as "tic douloureux", is a type of chronic pain affecting the trigeminal nerve. The trigeminal nerve is the 5th and the biggest cranial nerve and is responsible for the sensation in the face and motor functions such as biting and chewing. The maxillary and mandibular branches of the trigeminal nerve are most affected. The maxillary branch offers sensory supply to the mucous membrane, skin, nasal cavity, maxillary sinus and cheeks, upper lip, the upper incisors, canines, premolars, molars, and the gingiva. The mandibular branch is both sensory and motor. It offers sensory supply to the lower lip, chin, mucous membranes, bottom area of the oral cavity, and the lower incisors, canines, premolars, molars, and the gingiva. It offers motor supply to the muscles of mastication. People who suffer from TN often describe the pain as a severe, sharp, stabbing and burning pain and usually affects one side of the face often triggered by a mild touch, speaking, chewing, brushing teeth, shaving, smiling or even just wind blowing on the cheek area.

Variants

There are 2 types of Trigeminal Neuralgia. Type 1 (TN1 or classic TN) and Type 2 (TN2 or atypical TN). TN1 is characterized by sudden, excruciating, extreme electric shock-like pain shooting through the face and usually lasts from a few seconds to several minutes, and occurs many times a day. However, in between episodes, the patient is completely free of pain. TN2 is characterized

trigeminal neuralgia
三叉神経痛

tic douloureux
疼痛性チック

cranial nerve　脳神経

nasal cavity　鼻腔

maxillary sinus
上顎洞

incisor　切歯

canine　犬歯

premolar　小臼歯

molar　臼歯

mastication　咀嚼

by a constant burning, crushing, aching pain that does not seem to go away. Treatments for both types are also different.

Etiology

TN is usually caused by a blood vessel impinging on the nerve, causing it to malfunction. Other known causes are tumors growing next to the nerve, damage to the myelin sheath, trauma to the face, surgical injuries, stroke, or simply because of aging.

impinging　圧迫する

malfunction
故障, 機能不全

tumor　腫瘍

myelin sheath
髄鞘, ミエリン鞘

stroke　脳卒中

Epidemiology

TN usually affects middle-aged women. The ratio of women and men who have TN is 3 to 1. Those in the age bracket between 37 and 67 years are the most affected (De Toledo IP, 2016). Additionally, there is evidence that the disorder can be hereditary. Hypertension and multiple sclerosis are also reported to be risk factors.

hereditary　遺伝性の

hypertension
高血圧

multiple sclerosis
多発性硬化症

Symptoms

TN is sometimes described by sufferers as the most excruciating pain known to humanity. The pain typically involves the lower face and jaw, although sometimes it affects the area around the nose and above the eye.

Differential Diagnosis

The most common way to diagnose TN is through the patient's symptoms and history. Magnetic resonance imaging (MRI) is usually used to check if tumors or blood vessels are impinging on the nerve but this has limitations. MRI may not be able to detect blood vessels that are deep or next to the nerve root. Examples of disorders that exhibit similar symptoms as TN are temporal tendinitis, which involves cheek pain and tooth sensitivity, as well as headaches and neck and shoulder pain. Another condition is occipital neuralgia, which involves pain in the front and back of the head that sometimes extends into the facial region. Different tests may be used with patient's reported symptoms to rule out other facial disorders.

temporal tendinitis
側頭筋腱炎

occipital neuralgia
後頭神経痛

rule out　除外する

Treatment

Treatment for TN is usually focused on alleviating the pain using medications and surgery. Commonly used medications are drugs that have anti-convulsant or muscle relaxant properties. These drugs can effectively control pain, but they also produce side effects and higher doses, which may be indicated in severe cases, may cause liver and kidney toxicity. If medications are ineffective, surgical treatment may be performed. Surgery is performed on the trigeminal nerve by treating a nearby blood vessel (microvascular decompression), thereby removing the underlying cause, and is thus often the treatment of choice for most patients.

alleviate　軽減する

anti-convulsant
抗けいれん薬

muscle relaxant
properties
筋弛緩作用

toxicity　毒性

microvascular
decompression
微小血管減圧

Exercise 5

T or F

If the following sentence is true mark T (true), if it is not true mark F (false).

1. ☐ Trigeminal Neuralgia (TN) is a disorder of the 5th branch of the cranial nerve.
2. ☐ Trigeminal Neuralgia is also known as Tn-syndrome.
3. ☐ TN affects men more than women.
4. ☐ TN is described as a severe pain that can easily be relieved by aspirin.
5. ☐ TN is caused by an artery putting pressure on the trigeminal nerve.

Sources：De Toledo IP, Conti Réus J, Fernandes M, Porporatti AL, Peres MA, Takaschima A, Linhares MN, Guerra E, De Luca Canto G). Prevalence of trigeminal neuralgia: A systematic review. J Am Dent Assoc. 2016 Jul;147(7):570-576.e2. doi: 10.1016/j.adaj.2016.02.014. Epub 2016 Mar 24.)

14 Paranasal Sinusitis

Dental Interview

Exercise 1   Listen to the dialogue and answer the following questions.

Interview questions

1. Why is Ms. Green calling a dental university?

   _____

2. Where exactly is the pain?

   _____

3. What kind of symptoms does she have?

   _____

4. What is maxillary sinusitis?

   _____

5. What is the occupation of Ms. Green?

   _____

Exercise 2

Listen to the dialogue and complete the following sentences.

Fill in the blanks

> G：Ms. Green, a 29-year-old flight attendant
>
> H：Dr. Hanaoka, an oral surgeon

At a dental university

The phone is ringing at 10:00 AM

H：Hello! This is Dr. Hanaoka speaking. May I help you?

G：Hi, I hope you can help. I have pain and a fever. Is it possible to get seen today?

H：Could you please describe your pain and where it is located?

G：I have a dull pain in my left cheek.

H：All right. Can you come to our university today?

G：Sure, I can.

3 PM

H：Good afternoon, Ms. Green! My name is Dr. Hanaoka and I'll be _____ you today. Could you please explain more precisely your problem?

G：I'm a flight attendant for British Airways. I think I might have caught a cold from a passenger on the international flight from London to Narita on the 2nd of January. Since the flight, I have been sick and have had a fever and pain. Although, I am taking pills for the common cold, these haven't helped me.

H：Sorry, before I examine you, I need to ask a few questions about your general health. Do you have any medical conditions or have you ever been _____?

G：I wasn't hospitalized, but I went to a dental clinic to _____ _____ my left upper wisdom tooth on the 27th of December last year. I had no problems after the treatment.

After the examination

H：Ms. Green, it looks like you have maxillary sinusitis.

G：What's that?

H：Maxillary sinusitis is _____ of the maxillary sinus. The symptoms of maxillary sinusitis can be fever, pain, pressure in the face near the cheekbones, toothache, and a runny _____. The maxillary sinus is one of the four sinuses, around the nose. These sinuses are called paranasal sinuses and are part of the upper airway, and are connected to the nasal cavity.

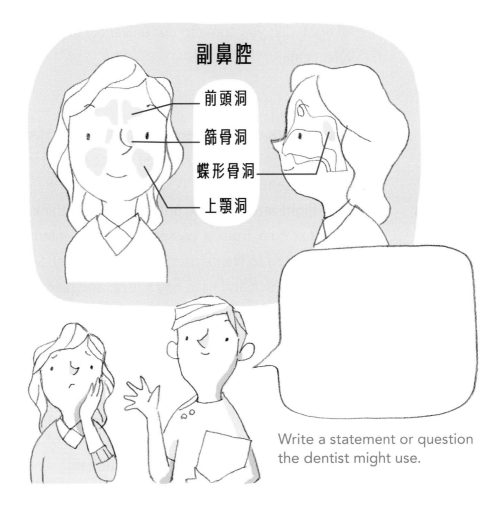

副鼻腔

前頭洞

篩骨洞

蝶形骨洞

上顎洞

Write a statement or question the dentist might use.

14 Paranasal Sinusitis

Read the dialogue and check the answers.

Learn the points

> G：Ms. Green, a 29-year-old flight attendant
>
> H：Dr. Hanaoka, an oral surgeon

At a dental university

The phone is ringing at 10:00 AM

H：Hello! This is Dr. Hanaoka speaking. May I help you?

G：Hi, I hope you can help. I have pain and a fever. Is it possible to get seen today?

H：Could you please describe your pain and where it is located?

G：I have a dull pain in my left cheek.

H：All right. Can you come to our university today?

G：Sure, I can.

3 PM

H：Good afternoon, Ms. Green! My name is Dr. Hanaoka and I'll be <u>treating</u> you today. Could you please explain more precisely your problem?

G：I'm a flight attendant for British Airways. I think I might have caught a cold from a passenger on the international flight from London to Narita on the 2nd of January. Since the flight, I have been sick and have had a fever and pain. Although, I am taking pills for the common cold, these haven't helped me.

H：Sorry, before I examine you, I need to ask a few questions about your general health. Do you have any medical conditions or have you ever been <u>hospitalized</u>?

G：I wasn't hospitalized, but I went to a dental clinic to <u>pull out</u> my left upper wisdom tooth on the 27th of December last year. I had no problems after the treatment.

After the examination

H：Ms. Green, it looks like you have maxillary sinusitis.

G：What's that?

H：Maxillary sinusitis is <u>inflammation</u> of the maxillary sinus. The symptoms of maxillary sinusitis can be fever, pain, pressure in the face near the cheekbones, toothache, and a runny <u>nose</u>. The maxillary sinus is one of the four sinuses, around the nose. These sinuses are called paranasal sinuses and are part of the upper airway, and are connected to the nasal cavity.

 Key words in the dialogue

dull pain：鈍い痛み
maxillary sinusitis：上顎洞炎
symptoms：症状
runny nose：鼻水
maxillary sinus：上顎洞
paranasal sinuses：副鼻腔
nasal cavity：鼻腔

Exercise 4

Let's learn some useful phrases.

Phrases to memorize

1. My name is Dr. Hanaoka and I'll be treating you today.
   本日，担当の花岡です．

2. Could you please describe your pain and where is it located?
   どこが痛むのかくわしく話していただけますか．

3. Could you please explain more precisely your problem?
   病状をもう少しくわしく説明していただけますか．

Reading 14

Paranasal Sinusitis

Paranasal Sinusitis

Sinusitis is inflammation of the upper respiratory tract and is prevalent in otorhinolaryngological practice. The paranasal sinuses are hollow spaces surrounding the nasal cavity, comprising of the frontal, ethmoid, sphenoid, and maxillary sinuses. Sinusitis commonly manifests as empyema and is usually of nasal origin; however, approximately 10% of maxillary sinusitis cases are attributable to infections of dental origin.

Definition of Maxillary Sinusitis

The maxillary sinus is comparatively small at birth and becomes deeper and broader as the permanent teeth erupt. It attains the normal adult size at around 15 years of age, when the eruption of the second molars is complete. Therefore, there is only a small distance separating the roots of the maxillary molars from the maxillary sinus, and inflammation can readily spread from suppurative apical lesions of these roots to the sinus. Particularly, the maxillary first molar most often contributes to the development of infection, which can manifest as either acute odontogenic maxillary sinusitis or chronic odontogenic maxillary sinusitis. Here, we will discuss chronic odontogenic maxillary sinusitis.

Chronic Odontogenic Maxillary Sinusitis

Chronic odontogenic maxillary sinusitis can be chronic from its onset itself or a case of acute odontogenic maxillary sinusitis that has become chronic. Clinical symptoms include unilateral headache, heavy-headedness, nasal congestion, post-nasal discharge, purulent nasal discharge, olfactory abnormalities, and/

paranasal sinusitis
副鼻腔炎

respiratory tract
気道

otorhinolaryngological
耳鼻咽喉科

nasal cavity　鼻腔

frontal sinus　前頭洞

ethmoid sinus
篩骨洞

sphenoid sinus
蝶形骨洞

maxillary sinus
上顎洞

empyema　蓄膿症

suppurative apical lesions
化膿した根尖部

odontogenic　歯性

onset　発症

nasal congestion
鼻づまり

purulent　化膿した

olfactory　嗅覚

or dull pain in the infraorbital region. Systemic symptoms and local symptoms of chronic sinusitis are minor compared to that of acute maxillary sinusitis. Discomfort or percussion pain is often observed with the causative tooth.

Radiographic imaging or computed tomography (CT) can be used. Radiographs show diffuse opacity in the maxillary sinus on the affected side, while CT images show thickening of the mucosa of the maxillary sinus.

Treatment comprises of extraction of the causative tooth or removal of the periapical lesion, and administration of antibiotics or anti-inflammatory agents. If possible, sinus lavage is also indicated. Radical maxillary sinus operation is considered when the aforementioned conservative treatment has no marked effect, or when there is frequent recurrence. Radical maxillary sinus operation involves the removal of the diseased sinus mucosa and creation of a counter-opening in the inferior nasal meatus. Surgical methods include the Caldwell-Luc approach and Watsuji-Denker approach. It should be remembered that this is an odontogenic condition presenting with nasal symptoms.

infraorbital　眼窩下

percussion　打診

mucosa　粘膜

periapical lesion
歯根尖周囲

sinus lavage
上顎洞洗浄

recurrence　再発

counter-opening
対孔形成

inferior nasal meatus
下鼻道

Exercise 5

T or F

If the following sentence is true mark T (true), if it is not true mark F (false).

1. ____ The paranasal sinuses consist of three sinuses.
2. ____ 90% of maxillary sinusitis cases are rhinologic.
3. ____ Post-nasal discharge is a symptom of maxillary sinusitis.
4. ____ Diagnosis by X-ray imaging is impossible.
5. ____ Surgical intervention is necessary when no improvement with pharmacotherapy is observed.

14 Paranasal Sinusitis

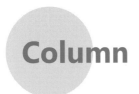

Column

上顎洞炎 —やや専門的に—

　歯性上顎洞炎は鼻性と異なり，歯に由来した上顎洞炎を総称するものです．したがって，歯周疾患やう蝕症に継発した根尖病変，歯内療法時や侵襲的歯科治療に起因した上顎洞穿孔，歯根やインプラント体の洞内迷入によって生じるものがこれにあたります．近年，インプラント治療が普及し，一般開業医が上顎洞に外科的侵襲を加えることが，以前と比較すると増加傾向にあり，そのため上顎洞が歯科医師全体にとってさらに身近な存在となっていることは言うまでもありません．

　上顎洞炎は耳鼻咽喉科において経験頻度の高い疾病であり，「急性副鼻腔炎診療ガイドライン」が日本鼻科学会から発刊されています．しかしながら，歯性上顎洞炎については急性鼻副鼻腔炎と病態や治療法が異なるとされ，収載されていないのが現状です．

　通常，上顎洞内は上顎洞粘膜で裏層されています．その上顎洞粘膜は線毛上皮であり，洞内に侵入した細菌や粉塵は重力に逆らうように中鼻道に開口している自然孔より排出されます．上顎洞内に迷入した歯根の一部が自然排出したとの話を聞いたことがあります．それは，線毛機能が正常であれば自然孔への排出運動が非常に活発であることの例えなのかもしれません．

　歯性上顎洞炎の治療は，抗菌療法と原因歯の治療による保存的治療が第一選択です．しかし，改善が認められない難治療例では上顎洞根治術が適応とされます．一般的には犬歯窩よりアプローチする Caldwel-Luc 法が用いられることが多くあります．ある程度の骨を除去し，上顎洞内の粘膜を剥離摘出しますが，上顎洞上方部は直視が困難であることが多くあります．近年ではCTやMRIなどの画像データ上で現在の操作部位を示す，ナビゲーションシステムを用いた取り組みもなされています．コンピュータの３次元位置測定・表示能力を，手術時に活用するコンピュータ支援外科は他領域において以前より使用されています．1970年代より Caldwel-Luc 法においてファイバースコープを用い，直視困難な上顎洞上方部の観察が行われており，直視不可能な手術部位の確認が可能になる反面，広視野で術野を確認することは困難であり，重大な損傷を伴う危険性もあります．ナビゲーションシステムは内視鏡下副鼻腔手術に多く応用されており，より安全な手術が可能であると報告されています．口腔外科領域においてさらなる普及が望まれています．

Column (English translation)

Odontogenic maxillary sinusitis is a blanket term for maxillary sinusitis of dental origin, as opposed to sinusitis of nasal origin. Therefore, this includes conditions caused by periapical lesions due to periodontal disease or dental caries, maxillary sinus perforation caused during endodontic treatment or by invasive dental treatment, and accidental insertion of a dental root or an implant into the maxillary sinus. With the recent spread of implant treatment, invasive surgery in the maxillary sinus by general practitioners has increased. Thus, it is understood that the members of the dental profession are becoming more familiar with the maxillary sinus as a whole.

Maxillary sinusitis cases are frequent in the field of otorhinolaryngology, and the Japanese Rhinologic Society has published the "Guidelines for the diagnosis and treatment of acute sinusitis." However, odontogenic maxillary sinusitis differs in its presentation and treatment protocol from acute sinusitis. It is currently not mentioned in the guidelines.

Ordinarily, the inside of the maxillary sinus is lined with maxillary sinus mucosa. The maxillary sinus mucosa consists of ciliated epithelium, and bacteria and dust invading the sinus are expelled, as if to defy gravity, from the natural pores opening into the middle nasal meatus. In some cases, it has been suggested that the dental roots entering the maxillary sinus are ejected naturally. This is clearly an example of the very active movement due to normal ciliary function to bring about expulsion from the natural ostia.

Regarding the treatment of odontogenic maxillary sinusitis, conservative treatment with antimicrobial therapy and treatment of the causative tooth is the first-line approach. However, radical maxillary sinus operation is deemed more suitable for refractive cases where no improvement is observed. Generally, the Caldwell-Luc approach from the canine fossa, is often used. A certain amount of bone is removed, and the mucosa within the maxillary sinus is detached and removed; however, in most cases, it is difficult to see the upper region of the maxillary sinus directly. Recently, navigation systems have been incorporated wherein the current treatment site is viewed using the imaging data from CT, magnetic resonance imaging. Computer-supported surgery, where the three-dimensional positional measurement and display capacity of a computer is actively used during surgery, has been used for some time in other fields. Since the 1970s, a fiberscope has been used in the Caldwell-Luc approach to observe the upper region of the maxillary sinus, which is difficult to see directly. However, it is difficult to confirm the surgical field within a broad visual field even though it becomes possible to confirm surgical sites that cannot be viewed directly, and there is the risk of serious damage. Navigation systems are frequently applied in endoscopic sinus surgery, and they reportedly enable safer operations; therefore, their use in the field of oral and maxillofacial surgery is desirable.

参考文献：白砂兼光・古郷幹彦編著：口腔外科学 第 3 版，医歯薬出版，2010
野間弘康・瀬戸院一監修：標準口腔外科学 第 4 版，医学書院，2015
日本鼻科学会：急性鼻副鼻腔炎診療ガイドライン 2010 年版，2014
阿知波基信，井上博貴，竹本隆：上顎洞根治術に対するナビゲーションシステムの使用経験，愛知学院大学歯学誌 52 502-506,2014

Case Report

15

1 Periodontal disease

A 74-year-old man visited a dental university with a chief complaint of swollen gums that covered his teeth. He had no pain and had started taking medication for hypertension for 5 years. A medical interview, periodontal pocket examination and X-rays revealed a diagnosis of drug-induced gingival overgrowth.

The dentist contacted his physician and had him change his medicine for hypertension. The dentist instructed the patient to brush his teeth and provided dental cleaning. Then, periodontal surgery was performed on the areas of significant swelling.

After the surgery, his periodontal condition recovered and he has been maintaining his oral health through regular visits to the dentist's office.

chief complaint
主訴

drug-induced gingival overgrowth
薬物性歯肉増殖症

2 Toothache

A 67-year-old woman presented to a dental office with a chief complaint of chewing pain and pus draining from the fistula near her maxillary left second molar. She had been treated for caries six months before, but left it untreated in the process. She has been aware of the pain for a week. After examination, he diagnosed her with periapical periodontitis and underwent infected root canal treatment.

This treatment has been successfully completed and she is now able to chew without problems with the tooth that has been crowned.

chewing pain
咬合痛

pus draining
排膿

fistula
瘻孔

periapical periodontitis
根尖性歯周炎

3 Herpes simplex

27-year-old female. She visited the dental hospital with a chief complaint of pain and vesicles on the left upper lip. She had been aware of a tingling pain in her upper lip since the day before yesterday, and when she woke up this morning, a blister appeared on her upper lip. Once or twice a year for the past five years, she had recurrent episodes of similar blisters on her upper lip, which would lighten in about 7 to 10 days.

She was diagnosed with herpes labialis and prescribed antiviral medication and an ointment to be applied on her lips. She was also instructed to maintain a regular diet, as a weakened immune system increases the likelihood of recurrence of herpes labialis.

herpes labialis
口唇ヘルペス

likelihood
可能性

4 What would be your provisional diagnosis?

A 68-year old male patient visits your clinic complaining of toothache around his upper right back teeth. Except for his chief complaint, he does not have any other signs or symptoms of concern. During the course of the oral examination, you notice an occlusal cavity on the upper right 1st molar and decide to restore it. While performing restorative treatment, you notice a white patch along the right lateral border of the tongue. Upon careful examination, you notice that the surface showed a cracked mud appearance and on palpation, it was raised and rough. The lesion was not tender to touch and not scrapable by cotton or dental instruments. You also noticed that the lips, buccal mucosa, pharynx, and extra oral soft tissues appeared normal and lymphadenopathy was absent. You continue and finish the tooth restoration and invite the patient for further discussion. During the interview, you gather the following information:

1. No systemic diseases
2. No serious medical problems
3. Not taking any medications other than vitamins and supplements
4. No sharp teeth that could possibly cause trauma to the affected area (tongue)
5. Not wearing dentures
6. Blood tests are normal
7. Heavy smoker but does not chew tobacco
8. Lymph nodes are not swollen

What would be your provisional diagnosis?

occlusal cavity
咬合面う蝕

on palpation　触診で

buccal mucosa
頬粘膜

pharynx　咽頭

lymphadenopathy
リンパ節腫脹

Lymph nodes
リンパ節

Leukoplakia

5 What would be your provisional diagnosis?

A 61-year-old woman presented to her general dentist with a complaint of pain associated with the maxillary left first premolar. The patient described a sharp, lancing pain that was triggered by stimulation of the tooth in question. She also reported 2 specific episodes in which she experienced severe, shooting electrical shock-like pain followed by a hot sensation in the same area. One of these episodes was triggered by a cool breeze on her face and the other occurred while washing her face. Examination and radiographic assessment revealed a periapical osseous lesion resulting in a diagnosis of acute apical periodontitis. Nonsurgical endodontics was completed with no undue effects. Approximately 2 months after the endodontic treatment, the patient began to have a recurrence of the paroxysmal sharp, shooting pain with a marked increase in the frequency of these episodes. The pain was triggered by light touch of the left cheek. Each episode lasted 1 to 2 seconds; however, she occasionally had 5 to 10 repetitive bursts.

What would be your provisional diagnosis? What test/s would you like to do?

lancing　刺すような

recurrence　再発

paroxysmal
発作性の

Sources：Spencer C.J. The Journal of Pain, Vol 9, No 9 (September), 2008: pp 767-770), Mayo Clinic.org, aans. org, kenhub.com

Trigeminal Neuralgia

① 組み合わせで誤っているのはどれか．1つ選べ．

a 切　歯 ―――― incisor

b 犬　歯 ―――― canine

c 小臼歯 ――― premolar

d 智　歯 ――― impacted tooth

e 乳　歯 ――― deciduous tooth

(103回A-27)

② 英語で診断を意味するのはどれか．1つ選べ．

a analysis

b diagnosis

c treatment

d examination

e consultation

(104回C-34)

③ Gingivitis is （　　） caused by dental plaque.

（　　）に入るのはどれか．1つ選べ．

a aging

b tumor

c trauma

d malnutrition

e inflammation

(105回A-10)

④ Recent studies have shown that （　　） may be one of the most significant risk factors in the development and progression of periodontal disease.

（　　）に入るのはどれか．1つ選べ．

a smoking

b hypertension

c sugar intake

d heart disease

e lack of exercise

(106回A-6)

⑤ WHO の「健康」を定義する文章を示す．

"Health is a state of complete physical, （　　） and social well-being and not merely the absence of disease or infirmity.

（　　）に入るのはどれか．1つ選べ．

a dental

b mental

c medical

d chemical

e biological

(107回C-1)

⑥ The goal of （　　） is to explain the physical and chemical factors that are responsible for the origin, development, and progression of life.

（　　）に入るのはどれか．1つ選べ．

a pedodontics

b periodontology

c physiology

d prosthodontics

e psychology

(108回A-1)

⑦ A porcelain veneer is bonded to the （　　） surface of an anterior tooth to solve esthetic problems.

（　　）に入るのはどれか．1つ選べ．

a distal

b labial

c lingual

d mesial

e occlusal

(109回A-1)

⑧ Avoiding the frequent intake of fermentable carbohydrates, especially sucrose, in diets is important for the (　　) of early childhood caries.
（　　）に入るのはどれか．1つ選べ．

a treatment
b prevention
c restoration
d development
e decalcification

(110回A-10)

⑨ ALARA is an acronym for "As (　　) As Reasonably Achievable", which is a safety principle based on the minimization of radiation.
（　　）に入るのはどれか．1つ選べ．

a Low
b Large
c Level
d Liable
e Likely

(111回D-13)

⑩ Tooth erosion is defined as the irreversible loss of tooth structure due to exposure to (　　).
（　　）に入るのはどれか．1つ選べ．

a acids
b bacteria
c carbohydrates
d fluorides
e saliva

(111回A-17)

⑪ (　　) is the process of enabling people to increase control over, and to improve, their health.
（　　）に入るのはどれか．1つ選べ．

a Quality of life
b Health promotion
c Health assessment
d Population strategy
e Primary health care

(112回D-2)

⑫ Seaweed-derived (　　) forms an elastic and hydrocolloid impression material through a chemical reaction.
（　　）に入るのはどれか．1つ選べ．

a agar
b alginate
c polyether
d zinc oxide eugenol
e polydimethylsiloxane

(112回C-8)

⑬ (　　) is a chronic disease caused by inherited and/or acquired deficiency in production of insulin by the pancreas, or by the ineffectiveness of the insulin produced.
（　　）に入るのはどれか．1つ選べ．

a Hepatitis
b Periodontitis
c Osteoporosis
d Diabetes mellitus
e Myocardial infarction

(113回D-3)

⑭ (　　) reduce neural activities by blocking voltage-dependent Na^+ channels.
（　　）に入るのはどれか．1つ選べ．

a Antibacterial agents
b Local anesthetics
c Muscle relaxants
d Narcotic analgesics
e Nonsteroidal anti-inflammatory drugs

(113回C-5)

⑮ ( ), the study of the distribution and determinants of health-related states and events in specified populations, is a potent scientific tool to confront a new infectious disease.

（ ）に入るのはどれか．1つ選べ．

a Anatomy

b Biochemistry

c Epidemiology

d Pharmacology

e Physiology

（114回D-7）

⑯ The ( ) is a statement in the patient's own words of the subjective symptoms that motivated the patient to visit a dental clinic.

（ ）に入るのはどれか．1つ選べ．

a diagnosis

b medication

c family history

d chief complaint

e medical history

（115回D-10）

正答 ① d ② b ③ e ④ a ⑤ b
　　 ⑥ c ⑦ b ⑧ b ⑨ a ⑩ a
　　 ⑪ b ⑫ b ⑬ d ⑭ b ⑮ c
　　 ⑯ d

Appendix
Academic Terms
おさえておきたい歯科学術用語

◆歯種	Tooth type
永久歯	permanent teeth
切歯	incisors
	front teeth
中切歯	central incisor
側切歯	lateral incisor
犬歯	canine
	cuspid
臼歯	molars
小臼歯	premolar
	bicuspid teeth
第一小臼歯	first premolar
第二小臼歯	second premolar
大臼歯	molar
第一大臼歯	first molar
第二大臼歯	second molar
第三大臼歯・智歯	third molar
	wisdom tooth
乳歯	deciduous teeth
	milk teeth
乳切歯	deciduous incisor
	milk incisor
乳中切歯	deciduous central incisor
乳側切歯	deciduous lateral incisor
乳犬歯	deciduous canine
乳臼歯	deciduous molars
第一乳臼歯	deciduous first molar
第二乳臼歯	deciduous second molar
切縁・切端	incisal edge

	incisal margin
咬合側	occlusal
唇側	labial
頬側	buccal
舌側	lingual
近心	mesial
遠心	distal
前方	anterior
後方	posterior
咬頭・咬頭頂	cusp
小窩	pit
裂溝	fissure
	groove
隆線	ridge
歯頸	cervical
歯冠	crown
歯根	root
エナメル質	enamel
象牙質	dentin
セメント質	cementum
歯髄	dental pulp
歯根膜	periodontal membrane
	periodontal ligament
歯根管	root canal
上顎歯	maxillary teeth
	upper teeth
下顎歯	mandibular teeth
	lower teeth

◆口腔領域の解剖	anatomy of oral region
口腔	oral
	oral cavity
口唇	lip
	labium
舌	tongue
	lingual
舌尖	lingual apex
	tongue tip
舌縁	lingual margin

	tongue edge	顎二腹筋前腹	anterior belly of digastric muscle
舌根	lingual radix	顎二腹筋後腹	posterior belly of digastric muscle
	base of tongue		
舌背	dorsum lingual	顎舌骨筋	mylohyoid muscle
	dorsum of tongue	茎状舌骨筋	stylohyoid muscle
口蓋	palate	オトガイ舌骨筋	geniohyoid muscle
軟口蓋	soft palate	舌骨下筋群	infrahyoid muscles
硬口蓋	hard palate	甲状舌骨筋	thyrohyoid muscle
口蓋垂	uvula	胸骨舌骨筋	sternohyoid muscle
歯肉・歯茎	gingiva	肩甲舌骨筋	omohyoid muscle
	gum	胸骨甲状筋	sternothyroid muscle
鼻腔	nasal cavity	舌筋	muscles of tongue
咽頭	pharynx		lingual muscle
上咽頭	nasopharynx	内舌筋	intrinsic muscles of tongue
中咽頭	oropharynx		
下咽頭	hypopharynx	外舌筋	extrinsic muscles of tongue
喉頭	larynx		
喉頭蓋	epiglottis	茎突舌筋	styloglossus muscle
喉頭蓋谷	epiglottic vallecula	舌骨舌筋	hyoglossus muscle
声帯	vocal chords	オトガイ舌筋	genioglossus muscle
気管	trachea	口蓋舌筋	palatoglossal muscle
	windpipe	神経	nerves
食道	esophagus	三叉神経	trigeminal nerve
食道入口部	esophageal orifice	眼神経	optic nerve
上顎骨	maxilla	上顎神経	maxillary nerve
下顎骨	mandible	下顎神経	mandibular nerve
口蓋骨	palatine bone	顔面神経	facial nerve
側頭骨	temporal bone	迷走神経	vagus nerve
舌骨	hyoid bone	舌下神経	hypoglossal nerve
甲状軟骨	thyroid cartilage	唾液腺	salivary glands
咀嚼筋	masticatory muscle	大唾液腺	major salivary gland
咬筋	masseter	耳下腺	parotid gland
内側翼突筋	medial pterygoid muscle	顎下腺	submandibular gland
外側翼突筋	lateral pterygoid muscle	舌下腺	sublingual gland
		小唾液腺	miner salivary glands
側頭筋	temporal muscle		
舌骨上筋群	suprahyoid muscle	◆学習科目	**Learning Subject**
顎二腹筋	digastric muscle	歯科学	dentistry

歯学	odontology
口腔科学	stomatology
解剖学	anatomy
組織学	histology
生理学	physiology
病理学	pathology
薬理学	pharmacology
微生物学	microbiology
細菌学	bacteriology
衛生学	hygiene
口腔衛生学	oral health
社会歯科学	community dentistry
生化学	biochemistry
歯科理工学	dental materials and devices
口腔外科学	oral and maxillofacial surgery
歯科保存学	conservative dentistry
保存修復学	operative dentistry
歯内療法学	endodontology endodontics
歯周病学	periodontology
歯周治療学	periodontics
う蝕学	cariology
歯科補綴学	prosthetic dentistry prosthodontics
義歯学	denture prosthodontics
歯冠補綴架工義歯学	crown and bridge prosthodontics
小児歯科学	pediatric dentistry pedodontics
歯科矯正学	orthodontics
高齢者歯科学	geriatric dentistry
歯科麻酔学	dental anaesthesiology
障害者歯科学	special needs dentistry dentistry for disabled
歯科放射線学	dental radiology
口腔診断学	oral diagnostics

総合歯科学	general dentistry
口腔インプラント学	dental Implantology

◆歯科診療	**Dental practice**
全部床義歯（総義歯）	full denture complete denture
部分床義歯（局部床義歯）	partial denture
インレー	inlay
アンレー	onlay
クラウン（冠）	crown
ブリッジ（架工義歯）	bridge
口腔インプラント	oral implant
う蝕（むし歯）	caries dental caries
歯周病	periodontal disease
歯肉炎	gingivitis
歯周炎	periodontitis
歯髄炎	pulpitis
慢性	chronic
急性	acute
痛み（疼痛）	pain ache
咀嚼	mastication chewing
咬合	occlusion
不正咬合	malocclusion
嚥下	deglutition swallowing
嚥下障害	dysphasia swallowing disorder
疾患	disease
炎症	inflammation
腫脹	swelling
発赤	reddening
機能障害	dysfunction
膿瘍	abscess
口腔乾燥	dry mouth
口腔乾燥症	xerostomia

Appendix
Glossary of Dental Terms for CMED

A

Abrasion	The wearing out of tooth surfaces caused by mechanical force or pressure like excessive brushing of teeth. [related terms: attrition, erosion]
Abscess	A localized inflammation due to a collection of pus in the bone or soft tissue and is usually caused by an infection.
Abutment	A natural, stable, and healthy tooth used to support a prosthesis or denture.
Acrylic resin	A resinous material of various esters of acrylic acid that is used as denture base materials, dental restorations, and dental trays.
Acute	An illness or condition that develops quickly, is intense or severe and lasts a relatively short period of time. [related term: chronic]
Allergy	A condition in which exposure to a substance, such as pollen, latex, animal dander, or a particular food or drug, causes an overreaction by the immune system that results in symptoms such as sneezing, itching, rash, and difficulty breathing or swallowing.
Amalgam	A dental filling material, composed of mercury and other minerals, used to fill decayed teeth.
Analgesic	An agent or drug to lessen or relieve pain sensation without causing loss of consciousness. [related terms: painkiller, pain reliever]
Anesthesia	A loss of sensation with or without loss of consciousness.
Anesthetic	A class of drugs that eliminates or reduces pain especially during surgery.
Anterior (dental)	Refers to the incisor and canine teeth, tissues, and surfaces located towards the front of the mouth. [related term: posterior]
Appliance	A device used in dentistry to repair teeth or replace missing teeth and provide a functional or therapeutic effect.
Artery	A type of blood vessel that carries blood high in oxygen content away from the heart to the farthest reaches of the body. [related term: vein]
Attrition	The wearing out of tooth surfaces caused by excessive tooth-to-tooth contact caused by grinding, clenching, or developmental defects. It also occurs as a physiological process due to aging. [related terms: abrasion, erosion]

B

Benign	A condition, tumor, or growth that is not cancerous and does not invade surrounding tissues or spread to other parts of the body. [related term: malignant]
Bicuspid	A two-cusp tooth found between the molar and the canine. It is also known as the premolar tooth. [related term: premolar]
Biopsy	A process of removing tissue to determine the presence of pathology.
Bitewing X-ray	A type of radiographic photograph of the crowns of teeth to check for decay.
Bleaching	The technique of applying a chemical agent to the teeth to whiten them.
Bleeding	The escape of blood from an injured or ruptured blood vessel.
Bonding	A process to chemically attach composite filling material, veneers, or plastic/acrylic to the tooth's enamel.
Bridge	A fixed prosthetic replacement of one or more missing teeth cemented or attached to the abutment teeth or implant abutments adjacent to the space.
Bruxism	The involuntary clenching or grinding of the teeth.
Buccal	A surface or term of direction which denotes an area or point of the outer surface of the tooth that faces the cheek. [related terms: facial, labial, lingual, palatal, mesial, distal, occlusal]

C

Calculus	The hard deposit of mineralized plaque that forms on the crown and/or root of the tooth. Also referred to as tartar.
Candidiasis	A fungal infection caused by a species of yeast called Candida, usually Candida albicans, and is characterized as white patches on the tongue, or other areas of the mouth and throat. It is also called as oral thrush or moniliasis.
Canine	The third tooth from the midline located between the lateral incisor and first premolar, commonly called the eye tooth. [related terms: cuspids, incisors, premolars, molars]
Caries	A technical term for tooth decay. It is the progressive breaking down or dissolving of tooth structure, caused by the acid produced when bacteria digest sugars. [related terms: cavity, decay]
Cavity	A layman's term for tooth decay. Its dental term is caries or dental caries. It is also the dental term for the hole that is left after the decay has been removed (for example, cavity preparation). [related terms: caries, decay]
Cement	A special type of glue used to hold a crown in its place. It also acts as an insulator to protect the tooth's nerve.
Cementum	The very thin, bonelike structure that covers the root of the tooth. [related terms: enamel, dentin, pulp]
Chronic	An illness or condition that is continuing or occurring again and again for a long period of time. [related term: acute]

Clasp	A part of a removable partial denture that acts as a direct retainer or stabilizer for the denture by partially surrounding an abutment tooth.
Composite resin	A tooth-colored filling material made of plastic resin or porcelain.
Consultation	A diagnostic service provided by a dentist other than the treating dentist.
Cosmetic dentistry	Any dental treatment or repair that is solely rendered to improve the appearance of the teeth or mouth.
Crown (denture)	A dental restoration that covers the entire tooth and restores it to its original shape and function.
Crown (tooth)	The portion of a tooth that is covered by enamel. [related term: root]
Curettage	A deep scaling of that portion of the tooth below the gum line. Its purpose is to remove calculus and infected gum tissue.
Cusp	The protruding portion of a tooth's chewing surface.
Cuspid	A one-cusp tooth found between the incisors and the premolars. [related term: canine]

D

Decay	A layman's term for dental caries. It is the progressive breaking down or dissolving of tooth structure, caused by the acid produced when bacteria digest sugars. [related terms: caries, cavity]
Deciduous teeth	Are the first set of teeth in the growth and development of humans and most mammals. It is also called primary teeth, and informally known as baby teeth, milk teeth, or temporary teeth.
Dental fear	A severe type of anxiety and is a normal emotional reaction to one or more specific threatening stimuli in the dental situation. These stimuli can include fear of dental procedures, dental environment, dental instruments, or fear of the dentist as a person. It is also called dental phobia or dentophobia.
Dental hygienist	A dental professional specializing in cleaning the teeth by removing plaque, calculus, and oral health education.
Dentin	The part of the tooth that is under both the enamel which covers the crown and the cementum which covers the root. [related terms: enamel, cementum, pulp]
Dentition	The collective name of all teeth in the dental arch.
Denture	A removable appliance used to replace teeth. A complete denture replaces all the upper teeth and/or all the lower teeth.
Diabetes	A chronic disease in which the body's ability to produce or respond to the hormone insulin is impaired, resulting in abnormal metabolism of carbohydrates and elevated levels of glucose in the blood and urine.
Diagnosis	The identification of the nature of an illness or other problem by examination of the signs and symptoms. [related term: prognosis]
Diastema	A space between two adjacent teeth in the same dental arch.
Direct pulp capping	The procedure in which the exposed pulp is covered with a dressing or cement to protect the pulp and promote healing and repair.

Appendix

Distal	A surface or term of direction which denotes an area or point farther from any part of reference. [related terms: facial, buccal, labial, lingual, palatal, mesial, occlusal]
Dry socket	A localized inflammation of the tooth socket following an extraction due to infection and lack of formation of a blood clot. It is often caused by smoking or excessive rinsing after an extraction. It is also called osteitis.

E

Enamel	The hard, calcified portion of the tooth which covers the crown. The enamel is the hardest substance in the human body. [related terms: dentin, cementum, pulp]
Endodontic treatment	Treatment that deals with injuries to or diseases of the pulp, or nerve, of the tooth.
Erosion	A chemical process characterized by acid dissolution of dental hard tissue not involving acids of bacterial origin. [related terms: abrasion, attrition]
Erythroplakia	Are abnormal red lesions on the mucous membranes in the mouth that typically occur on the tongue or on the floor of the mouth and cannot be scraped off. They often indicate a precancerous condition. [related term: leukoplakia]
Extraction	The removal of a tooth from its socket. It is also known as exodontia.
Extraoral	Concerning the outside of the mouth. [related term: intraoral]

F

Facial	A surface or term of direction which denotes an area or point pertaining to or toward the face. Subdivision of the term includes buccal and labial. [related term: buccal, labial, lingual, palatal, mesial, distal, occlusal]
Facial nerve	Each of the seventh pair of cranial nerves that supply motor fibers to the muscles of the face and jaw and sensory and parasympathetic fibers to the tongue, palate, and fauces of the mouth.
Facial palsy	The temporary paralysis or weakness of the facial muscles affecting one eyelid and one side of the forehead and mouth.
Filling	A dental material used to fill a tooth cavity or replace part of a tooth.
Fissure	A deep ditch or cleft in the surface of the teeth. [related term: pit]
Floss	A thin, nylon string, waxed or unwaxed, that is inserted between the teeth to remove food and plaque.
Fluoride	A chemical compound used to prevent dental decay, utilized in fluoridated water systems and/or applied directly to the teeth.
Fracture (tooth)	A break or crack in the hard shell of the tooth commonly caused by trauma or excessive occlusal forces during biting or chewing.

G

General anesthesia	A combination of medications that put you in a sleep-like state before a surgery or other medical procedure. [related terms: local anesthesia, topical anesthesia]

Gingiva	The part of the oral mucosa covering the tooth-bearing border of the jaw. [related term: gums]
Gingivectomy	Removal of excessive gingiva. May be necessary to access tooth structure during a restorative procedure.
Gingivitis	An inflammation or infection of the gingiva; the initial stage of gum disease.
Gums	The part of the oral mucosa covering the tooth-bearing border of the jaw. [related term: gingiva]

H

Hairy Leukoplakia	An unusual form of leukoplakia that is seen only in people who are infected with HIV, have AIDS, or AIDS-related complex. The lesion cannot be scraped off and appears raised, with a corrugated or "hairy" surface, hence the name.
Halitosis	An oral health problem where the main symptom is bad smelling breath. It is commonly known as bad breath.
Handpiece (dental)	A hand-held, mechanical instrument used to perform a variety of common dental procedures, including removing decay, polishing fillings, performing cosmetic dentistry, and altering prostheses.
Hepatitis	The inflammation of the liver, caused by infectious or toxic agents and characterized by jaundice, fever, liver enlargement, and abdominal pain.
Herpes	Any of a group of viral diseases caused by herpes viruses, affecting the skin. It causes sores or blisters to form in or around the mouth or genitals.
HIV (Human Immunodeficiency Virus)	A virus that attacks the body's immune system. If HIV is not treated, it can lead to AIDS or acquired immunodeficiency syndrome.
Hypertension	A common condition in which the long-term force of the blood against your artery walls is high enough that it may eventually cause health problems, such as heart disease. It is commonly known as high blood pressure.

I

Immunity	The resistance of the body to infection by a disease-causing agent, such as bacteria or virus.
Impacted tooth	An unerupted or partially erupted tooth that is positioned against bone or soft tissue so that total eruption is unlikely.
Implant	An artificial device, usually make of a metal alloy or ceramic material, that is implanted within the jawbone to attach an artificial crown, denture, or bridge.
Impression (dental)	An imprint of the teeth and surrounding tissues, formed with a plastic material that hardens into a mold for use in making dentures, inlays, or plastic models.
Incidence	The number of cases of an event, such as a disease, occurring in a particular population during a given period. [related term: prevalence]

Incipient caries	Dental carries in an early stage of development, often not requiring immediate restorations.
Incisal	Pertaining to the cutting edges of incisor and cuspid teeth.
Incisors	Are the front teeth adapted for cutting and are located between the canines on both sides of the jaws. [related terms: canines, premolars, molars]
Indirect pulp capping	A procedure in which the nearly exposed pulp as covered with a protective dressing to protect the pulp from additional injury and to promote healing and repair via formation of secondary dentin.
Infection	The invasion and multiplication of microorganisms such as bacteria, viruses, and parasites that are not normally present within the body.
Inflammation	The body's natural reaction against injury and infection. Part of the body becomes reddened, swollen, hot, and often painful.
Injection	The act or an instance of injecting a drug or other substance into the body either under or through the skin or into the tissues, a vein, muscle, or a body cavity.
Injury	A damage inflicted on the body by an external force.
Inlay	A cast gold filling that is used replace part of the tooth. [related term: onlay]
Insurance	A contract that requires an insurer (private or public) to pay some or all of a person's healthcare costs in exchange for a premium.
Interproximal	The area or point between two adjacent teeth.
Intraoral	The inside of a mouth. [related term: extraoral]
J	
Jaundice	A medical condition with yellowing of the skin or whites of the eyes, arising from excess of the pigment bilirubin and typically caused by obstruction of the bile duct or by liver disease.
Jaw	A common name for either the maxilla or the mandible.
Joint	The point where two or more bones or a bone and a cartilage are attached to the body. Joints may be movable or fixed.
L	
Labial	A surface or term of direction which denotes an area or point pertaining to or around the lip. [related terms: facial, buccal, lingual, palatal, mesial, distal, occlusal]
Laceration	A deep cut or tear in skin or flesh due to trauma or injury. [related terms: rash, sore, ulcer]
Leukoplakia	Are thickened, white patches form on your gums, the insides of your cheeks, the bottom of your mouth and, sometimes, your tongue. These patches cannot be scraped off.
Lingual	A surface or term of direction which denotes an area or point pertaining to or around the tongue. [related terms: facial, buccal, labial, palatal, mesial, distal, occlusal]

Local anesthesia	An injection given in the mouth to numb the areas where a tooth or area needs a dental procedure. [related terms: general anesthesia, topical anesthesia]
Lymph nodes	Are oval-shaped masses of tissue in the body that serve an important role in protecting the body from infection and cancer.

M

Malaise	A condition of general bodily weakness or discomfort, often marking the onset of a disease.
Malignant	The term literally means growing worse and resisting treatment. In reference to a neoplasm or cancerous growth, it means having the properties of locally invasive and destructive growth and metastasis.
Malnutrition	Refers to deficiencies, excesses, or imbalances in a person's intake of energy and/or nutrients.
Malocclusion	The improper alignment of biting or chewing surfaces of upper and lower teeth.
Mandible	The technical term for the lower jaw. [related terms: jaw, maxilla]
Mastication	The act of chewing.
Maxilla	The technical term for the upper jaw. [related terms: jaw, mandible]
Mesial	A surface or term of direction which denotes an area or point toward or situated in the middle. [related terms: facial, buccal, labial, lingual, palatal, distal, occlusal]
Molars	Are the broad, multi-cusped back teeth, used for grinding food are considered the largest teeth in the mouth. There are a total of twelve molars, three on each side of the upper and lower jaws. [related terms: incisors, canines, premolars]
Morbidity	Refers to the incidence or prevalence of a disease in a specific population or location. [related term: mortality]
Mortality	Refers to the relative frequency of deaths in a specific population or location. [related term: morbidity]
Mucosa	The inner lining of the cheeks and lips, which is an anatomic region that includes all the mucous membrane lining of the inner surface of the cheeks and lips.

N

Nausea	A feeling of sickness in the stomach characterized by an urge to vomit.
Nitrous oxide	A controlled mixture of nitrogen and oxygen gases (N_2O) that is inhaled by the patient to decrease sensitivity to pain. Also referred to as laughing gas.
Numb/Numbness	The loss of feeling or sensation in an area of the body.

O

Obesity	An abnormal accumulation of body fat, usually 20% or more over an individual's ideal body weight.

Occlusal	A surface or term of direction which denotes an area or point pertaining to the chewing surface of the back teeth. [related terms: facial, buccal, labial, lingual, palatal, mesial, distal]
Occlusion	Any contact between biting or chewing surfaces of upper and lower teeth.
Odontogenic	Refers to the formation and development of teeth.
Onlay	A cast gold or porcelain filling that covers one or all of the tooth's cusps. [related term: inlay]
Onset	The first appearance of the signs or symptoms of an illness.
Oral cavity	A scientific and anatomical term for the inside of the mouth.
Oral hygiene	The practice of keeping the mouth clean and healthy by brushing and flossing to prevent tooth decay and gum disease.
Oral mucosa	The mucous membrane lining the inside surfaces of the mouth.
Oral thrush	A fungal infection caused by a species of yeast called Candida, usually Candida albicans, and is characterized as white patches on the tongue, or other areas of the mouth and throat. It is also called as candidiasis or moniliasis.
Orthodontics treatment	A treatment to correct malocclusion and restore the teeth to its proper alignment and function. A common orthodontic treatment is the use of braces.
Overbite	A condition in which the upper teeth excessively overlap vertically the lower teeth when the jaw is closed. [related terms: overjet, underbite]
Overjet	A condition in which the upper teeth excessively overlap horizontally the lower teeth when the jaw is closed. [related terms: overbite, underbite]
P	
Pain	A localized or generalized unpleasant bodily sensation that causes mild to severe physical discomfort and emotional distress and typically results from bodily disorder such as injury or disease.
Painkiller	An agent or drug to lessen or relieve pain sensation without causing loss of consciousness. It is also known as pain reliever. [related term: analgesic]
Palatal	A surface or term of direction which denotes an area or point facing or pertaining to the palate. [related terms: facial, buccal, labial, lingual, mesial, distal, occlusal]
Palate	The hard and soft tissues forming the roof of the mouth.
Palliative	A treatment that relieves pain but is not curative.
Panoramic X-ray or Panorex	An extraoral full-mouth X-ray that records the teeth and the upper and lower jaws on one film.
Partial denture	A removable appliance used to replace one or more lost teeth.
Pathology	The scientific study of the nature of disease and its causes, processes, development, and consequences.

Percussion	A method of tapping body parts with fingers, hands, or small instruments as part of a physical or medical examination.
Periapical	The area that surrounds the tip of a tooth root.
Periapical abscess	A collection of pus that occurs at the root tip due to bacterial infection.
Pericoronitis	An inflammation of the gum tissue around the crown of a tooth, usually the third molar.
Periodontal	Relating to the tissue and bone that supports the tooth (from *peri*, meaning around, and *dont*, meaning tooth).
Periodontal disease	The inflammation and infection of the gums, ligaments, bone, and other tissues surrounding the teeth. Gingivitis and periodontitis are the two main forms of periodontal disease.
Periodontal pocket	An abnormal deepening of the gingival crevice. It is caused when disease and infection destroy the ligament that attaches the gum to the tooth and the underlying bone.
Periodontal surgery	A surgical procedure involving the gums and jawbone. Intended to reduce periodontal disease.
Periodontist	The area of dentistry concerned with the prevention, diagnostic, and treatment of periodontal disease.
Periodontitis	Inflammation of the supporting structures of the tooth, including the gum, the periodontal ligament, and the jawbone.
Permanent teeth	The thirty-two adult teeth that replace the baby, or primary teeth. Also known as secondary teeth.
Phobia	An anxiety disorder characterized by extreme and irrational fear of simple things or social situations.
Pit	A recessed area found on the surface of a tooth, usually where the grooves of the teeth meet. [related term: fissure]
Plaque	A film of sticky material containing saliva, food particles, and bacteria that attaches to the tooth surface both above and below the gum line. When left on the tooth it can promote gum disease and decay.
Pontic	An artificial tooth used in a bridge to replace a missing tooth.
Posterior (dental)	Refers to the premolar and molar teeth, tissues, and surfaces located towards the back of the mouth. [related word: anterior]
Premolars	Refer to the back teeth (premolars and molars), tissues, and surfaces located towards the back of the mouth. Premolars are also known as bicuspids. [related terms: incisors, canines, molars]
Prescription	A written direction by a physician, dentist, or other health professionals for the preparation and use of a medicine or remedy.
Prevalence	The proportion of a population who have a specific characteristic in a given time period. [related term: incidence]
Primary teeth	The first set of teeth that humans get, lasting until the permanent teeth come in. [related terms: deciduous teeth, milk teeth, temporary teeth]
Prognosis	A medical prediction of the future course of a disease and the chance for recovery. [related term: diagnosis]

Appendix

Prophylaxis	The scaling and polishing procedure performed to remove calculus, plaque, and stains from the crowns of the teeth.
Prosthesis	Any device or appliance replacing one or more missing teeth.
Pulp	The hollow chamber inside the crown of the tooth that contains its nerves and blood vessels. [related terms: enamel, cementum, dentin]
Pulpectomy	The complete removal of the tooth's pulp. [related term: pulpotomy]
Pulpotomy	The partial removal of the tooth's pulp. [related term: pulpectomy]
Pus	A yellowish or green viscous fluid consisting of dead white blood cells, bacteria, and necrotic tissue.

Q

Quadrant	The dental term for the division of the jaws onto four parts, beginning at the midline of the arch and extending towards the last tooth in the back of the mouth. There are four quadrants in the mouth; each quadrant generally contains five to eight teeth.

R

Radiograph	An image produced on a sensitive plate or film by X-rays, gamma rays, or similar radiation, and typically used in medical examination.
Radiolucent	A material or tissue that allows passage of x-rays. Radiolucent structures are black or near black on conventional x-rays. [related term: radiopaque]
Radiopaque	A material or tissue that blocks passage of X-rays. Radiopaque structures are white or nearly white on conventional X-rays. [related term: radiolucent]
Rash	An area of redness and spots on a person's skin, appearing especially due to allergy or illness. [related terms: laceration, sore, ulcer]
Recur	To occur again or to return. For example, a symptom, sign, or disease can recur.
Referral	When a dental patient is sent to another dentist, usually a specialist, for treatment or consultation.
Reline	The process of resurfacing the tissue side of a denture with a base material.
Replantation	The return of a tooth to its socket.
Resorption	The breakdown and assimilation of the bone that supports the tooth. It is commonly known as bone loss.
Restoration	Any material or devise used to replace lost tooth structure (filling, crown) or to replace a lost tooth or teeth. For example: bridge, complete or partial dentures.
Retainer	A removable dental appliance, usually used in orthodontics, that maintains space between teeth or holds teeth in a fixed position until the bone solidifies around them.
Root	The part of the tooth below the crown, normally encased in the jawbone. It is made up of dentin, includes the root canal, and is covered by cementum. [related term: crown]

Root canal	The hollow part of the tooth's root. It runs from the tip of the root into the pulp.
Root canal therapy	The process of treating disease or inflammation of the pulp or root canal. This involves removing the nerves of the pulp and sealing it with medications and cement.
Root planing	The process of scaling and planing exposed root surfaces to remove all calculus, plaque, and infected tissue.
Rubber dam	A sheet of thin rubber used by dentists to isolate a tooth or teeth from the fluids of the mouth during dental treatment.

S

Saliva	A watery fluid that is secreted into the mouth by the salivary glands.
Scaling	A procedure used to remove plaque, calculus, and stains from the teeth.
Sealant	A composite material used to seal the decay-prone pits, fissures, and grooves of teeth to prevent decay.
Signs	An effect of a health problem that can be observed by someone else. Signs are objective things that can be seen, like a red spot on your skin. [related term: symptoms]
Sinus	A connected system of hollow cavities in the skull.
Sinusitis	An inflammation, or swelling, of the tissue lining the sinuses.
Socket	The hole in the jawbone in which the tooth fits.
Sore	An open skin lesion, wound, ulcer, source of pain, distress, or irritation. [related terms: laceration, rash, ulcer]
Space maintainer	A dental appliance that fills the space of a lost tooth or teeth and prevents the other teeth from moving into the space. Used especially in orthodontic and pedodontic treatment.
Splint/Splinting	A device or procedure used to fasten or stabilize teeth in the same dental arch to support them or to prevent or minimize movement.
Stainless steel crown	A pre-made metal crown, shaped like a tooth, that is used to temporarily cover a seriously decayed or broken-down tooth. Used most often on children's teeth.
Surgery	The treatment of injuries or diseases by cutting open the body and removing or repairing the damaged part.
Swelling	The transient abnormal enlargement of a body part or area due to fluid accumulation.
Symptoms	An effect noticed and experienced only by the person who has the condition. Symptoms are subjective and describe how a person feels. For example, pain and nausea. [related term: signs]
Syncope	The loss of consciousness resulting from insufficient blood flow to the brain. It is commonly known as fainting or passing out.
Systemic	Relating to the whole body.

Appendix

T

Tartar	The buildup of plaque that can form hard crusty deposits on the teeth and cause cavities. [related term: calculus]
Temporomandibular joint (TMJ)	The connecting hinge mechanism between the upper jaw and the base of the skull.
Third molar	The last of the three molar teeth, also called wisdom teeth. There are four 3rd molars, two in the lower jaw two in the upper jaw, on each side.
Tissues	An aggregation of similar cells or types of cells, together with any associated intercellular materials, adapted to perform one or more specific functions.
Toothache	Any pain or soreness within or around a tooth, indicating inflammation and possible infection.
Tooth decay	A layman's term for dental caries. It is the progressive breaking down or dissolving of tooth structure, caused by the acid produced when bacteria digest sugars. [related terms: caries, cavity, decay]
Topical anesthesia	A condition of temporary numbness caused by applying a substance directly to a surface of the body. [related terms: general anesthesia, local anesthesia]
Torus	A bony elevation of normal bone. Usually seen on the upper palate behind the front teeth or under the tongue inside the lower jaw.
Trauma	A psychological, emotional response to an event or an experience that is deeply distressing or disturbing.
Treatment	The use of an agent, procedure, or regimen, such as a drug, surgery, or exercise, to cure or mitigate a disease, condition, or injury.
Treatment plan	A list of work that the dentist proposes to perform on a dental patient based on the results of the x-rays, exam, and diagnosis. Often more than one treatment plan is presented.
Trigeminal nerve	Either of the fifth pair of cranial nerves, being the chief sensory nerve of the face and the motor nerve of the muscles of chewing and having both sensory and motor functions in the teeth, mouth, and nasal cavity.
Tumor	A new growth of tissue in which cell multiplication is uncontrolled and progressive.

U

Ulcer	An open sore of the skin, eyes or mucous membrane, often caused by an initial abrasion and generally maintained by an inflammation and/or an infection. [related terms: laceration, rash, sore]
Ultrasonic scaler	An ultrasonic instrument with a tip for supplying high-frequency vibrations, used to remove plaque and calculus from teeth.
Underbite	A type of malocclusion in which the lower jaw and its front teeth project beyond the upper front teeth. [related terms: overbite, overjet]

V

Vein	A type of blood vessel that brings blood from other parts of the body to the heart.
Veneer	An artificial filling material, usually plastic, composite, or porcelain, that is used to provide an aesthetic covering over the visible surface of a tooth. It is most often used on the front teeth.

W

Wisdom teeth	The third and final set of molars. [related term: third molar]

X

Xerostomia	The abnormal dryness of the mouth due to insufficient secretions, disease, or medications. It is commonly known as dry mouth.

Sources：ADA, Mayo Clinic, The Medical Dictionary

Appendix

Index

歯科学生のための医学英語 第2版
Comprehensive Medical English for Dentistry

2020 年 7 月 1 日　第 1 版第 1 刷発行
2023 年 3 月 1 日　第 2 版第 1 刷発行

編　　者　　影山　幾男

羽村　章

発 行 者　　百瀬　卓雄

発 行 所　　株式会社 学建書院

〒112－0004　東京都文京区後楽 1－1－15-3F
TEL (03) 3816-3888
FAX (03) 3814-6679
http://www.gakkenshoin.co.jp

表紙／イラストレーション　久保田　修康
印刷製本　シナノ印刷(株)

ISBN978-4-7624-1704-7